618 OCO (H)

Pl **Instant Work-Ups:**
A Clinical **Guide to Obstetric**
and Gynecologic Care

Instant Work-Ups:
A Clinical Guide to Obstetric and Gynecologic Care

Theodore X. O'Connell, MD

Program Director
Family Medicine Residency Program
Kaiser Permanente Woodland Hills
Woodland Hills, California
Assistant Clinical Professor
Department of Family Medicine
David Geffen School of Medicine at UCLA
Los Angeles, California
Partner Physician
Southern California Permanente Medical Group
Woodland Hills, California

Kathleen Dor, MD

Associate Program Director
Family Medicine Residency Program
Kaiser Permanente Woodland Hills
Woodland Hills, California
Clinical Instructor
Department of Family Medicine
David Geffen School of Medicine at UCLA
Los Angeles, California
Partner Physician
Southern California Permanente Medical Group
Woodland Hills, California

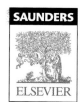

SAUNDERS

ELSEVIER

SAUNDERS
ELSEVIER

1600 John F. Kennedy Blvd.
Ste 1800
Philadelphia, PA 19103-2899

INSTANT WORK-UPS   ISBN: 978-1-4160-5461-0

Notice

Knowledge and best practice in this field are constantly changing. As new research
and experience broaden our knowledge, changes in practice, treatment and drug
therapy may become necessary or appropriate. Readers are advised to check the
most current information provided (i) on procedures featured or (ii) by the
manufacturer of each product to be administered, to verify the recommended
dose or formula, the method and duration of administration, and contraindications.
It is the responsibility of the practitioner, relying on their own experience and
knowledge of the patient, to make diagnoses, to determine dosages and the best
treatment for each individual patient, and to take all appropriate safety
precautions. To the fullest extent of the law, neither the Publisher nor the Authors
assumes any liability for any injury and/or damage to persons or property arising
out of or related to any use of the material contained in this book.

The Publisher

Library of Congress Cataloging-in-Publication Data

O'Connell, Theodore X.
Instant work-ups : a clinical guide to obstetric and gynecologic care / Theodore X.
O'Connell, Kathleen Dor. – 1st ed.
p. ; cm.
Includes bibliographical references.
ISBN 978-1-4160-5461-0
1. Obstetrics–Handbooks, manuals, etc. 2. Gynecology–Handbooks, manuals, etc.
I. Dor, Kathleen. II. Title. III. Title: Clinical guide to obstetric and gynecologic care.
[DNLM: 1. Genital Diseases, Female–Handbooks. 2. Gynecology–methods–Handbooks.
3. Obstetrics–methods–Handbooks. 4. Pregnancy Complications–Handbooks. WP 39
O18i 2009] RG531.O36 2009
618–dc22   2008020023

Acquisitions Editor: James Merritt
Developmental Editor: Greg Halbreich
Publishing Services Manager: Linda Van Pelt
Project Manager: Sharon Lee
Design Direction: Lou Forgione

Working together to grow
libraries in developing countries
www.elsevier.com | www.bookaid.org | www.sabre.org

ELSEVIER   BOOK AID International   Sabre Foundation

Printed in China
Last digit is the print number: 9   8   7   6   5   4   3   2   1

About the Authors

Theodore X. O'Connell, MD, is the Program Director of the Kaiser Permanente Woodland Hills Family Medicine Residency Program, where he also directs the residency research curriculum. Dr. O'Connell is a partner in the Southern California Permanente Medical Group and an assistant clinical professor in the Department of Family Medicine at the David Geffen School of Medicine at UCLA. He is the recipient of numerous clinical, teaching, and research awards. O'Connell has been published widely as the author of textbook chapters, review books, journal articles, and editorials. He received his medical degree from the University of California, Los Angeles School of Medicine and completed a residency and chief residency at Santa Monica-UCLA Medical Center in Santa Monica, California.

Kathleen Dor, MD, is the Associate Program Director of the Kaiser Permanente Woodland Hills Family Medicine Residency Program, where she directs the maternal-child health curriculum. Dr. Dor is a partner in the Soutern California Permanente Medical Group and a clinical instructor in the Department of Family Medicine at the David Geffen School of Medicine at UCLA. She received her medical degree from the University of California, Los Angeles School of Medicine and completed a residency and chief residency at Santa Monica-UCLA Medical Center.

For Sean
The most recent blessing for our family
Your smile is priceless.

Ted O'Connell

To Gil and Stephanie

Kathleen Dor

Foreword

The first ideas for this text came from our experiences as practicing clinicians involved in resident and medical student education. Most medical textbooks are oriented on the basis of a known diagnosis. If one wants to learn more about breast cancer, ectopic pregnancy, or medication use in pregnancy, traditional textbooks can be great sources of information.

However, patients do not come to the clinician labeled with a diagnosis, except for those problems that have been identified previously. Patients instead come with symptoms such as fatigue, postmenopausal vaginal bleeding, or galactorrhea. It is the role of the busy clinician to utilize the history, physical examination, and selected laboratory or imaging studies to sort out the patient's present symptom or laboratory abnormality and provide a diagnosis.

As we developed our clinical practice, we began creating lists of fairly standardized work-ups for common clinical problems. The work-up could then be tailored to each patient based upon history and physical exam findings. This process made it simpler to initiate work-ups, saved time in ordering these tests, and helped prevent forgetting any important components of the work-up.

Over time, we found that many of our residents were carrying our work-ups in their pockets for use with their patients, and that colleagues began using them as well. We began adding background information so that it would be clear why each test was indicated and in which cases additional portions of the work-up might be appropriate. Then one day it occurred to us that there were many more symptoms and clinical problems that could be outlined and explained in a similar format. Furthermore, many other busy clinicians might like to use these quick work-ups to save them time in their medical practices.

This text is directed to primary care physicians, but may be beneficial for physicians in almost all specialties. The work-ups outlined in each chapter are suggested courses of action based upon the current medical literature. However, they are not a replacement for clinical judgment and may not be uniformly applied to all patients. Every patient is different, and the history and physical examination may indicate a need for more or less evaluation than these work-ups suggest. These work-ups should be viewed as general guidelines to help the busy clinician be exacting and thorough while also being efficient. At the same time, deviating from these work-ups on the basis of clinical judgment is encouraged and expected.

We hope that this text eases your practice of medicine while helping you provide the highest quality care to your patients.

Ted O'Connell, MD
Kathleen Dor, MD

Table of Contents

1 | ABNORMAL PAP SMEAR (ABNORMAL CERVICAL CYTOLOGIC FINDINGS)

Kathleen Dor

Cervical cytology screening has significantly decreased rates of mortality from cervical cancer; however, 400 women die each year in the United States from cervical cancer, mostly as a result of inadequate screening.

Cervical cytology results are classified according to the Bethesda 2001 system (Box 1-1), which describes the categories of epithelial cell abnormalities. Histologic diagnoses of abnormalities are reported as cervical intraepithelial neoplasia (CIN) grades 1-3.

The glandular cell abnormalities are reported under the following categories: atypical glandular cells (AGC), subcategorized as endocervical, endometrial, or glandular not otherwise specified; AGC, favor neoplastic; endocervical adenocarcinoma in situ; and adenocarcinoma. Also noted are the presence of organisms, including *Trichomonas vaginalis* and fungal organisms morphologically consistent with *Candida* species; shift in flora suggestive of bacterial vaginosis; the presence of bacteria morphologically consistent with *Actinomyces* species; and cellular changes consistent with herpes simplex virus. Other findings that are noted include reactive cellular changes associated with inflammation, radiation, presence of intrauterine device, glandular cell status post hysterectomy, and atrophy.

In 2003, the U.S. Preventive Services Task Force recommended that all women be screened for cervical cancer with a cervical cytologic work-up beginning at age 21 or 3 years after sexual activity begins, whichever occurs first. Screening then should be performed at least every 3 years. Women who are older than 65 years need not undergo routine screening for cervical cancer if they have had appropriate screening and normal Pap smear results in the past. In addition, women who have had a total hysterectomy for a benign reason should not undergo screening for cervical cancer.

Most cases of cervical cancer are associated with infection with high-risk types of human papillomavirus (HPV) which are types 16, 18, 31, 33, 45, 51, 52, 56, 58, 5, 68, 73, and 82. HPV testing is used as an adjunct to the cervical cytologic work-up in women aged 30 years and older, as well as in cases of atypical squamous cells of undetermined significance (ASC-US) to determine whether a colposcopy should be performed.

Other risk factors for cervical cancer include cigarette smoking, immunocompromised status (e.g., human immunodeficiency virus [HIV] infection), early age at onset of sexual activity, multiple sexual partners, and sexual activity with male partners at high risk for sexually transmitted diseases.

Squamous Cell
- Atypical squamous cells (ASC)
  - Of undetermined significance (ASC-US)
  - Atypical squamous cells with high-grade intraepithelial lesion (ASC-H) cannot be ruled out
- Low-grade squamous intraepithelial lesions (LSIL)
  - Encompassing human papillomavirus (HPV), mild dysplasia, and cervical intraepithelial neoplasia (CIN) grade 1
- High-grade squamous intraepithelial lesions (HSIL)
  - Encompassing moderate and severe dysplasia, carcinoma in situ, CIN grade 2, and CIN grade 3
- Squamous cell carcinoma

Glandular Cell
- Atypical glandular cells (AGC)
- Atypical glandular cells, favor neoplastic
- Endocervical adenocarcinoma in situ
- Adenocarcinoma

Modified from Solomon D, Davey D, Kurman R, et al: The 2001 Bethesda System: terminology for reporting results of cervical cytology. Forum Group Members; Bethesda 2001 Workshop. JAMA 2002;287:2114-2119. Copyright © 2002, American Medical Association. All rights reserved.

Box 1-1. The 2001 Bethesda System Categorizing of Epithelial Cell Abnormalities

---

Medications That May Increase the Risk for Cervical Cancer

- Corticosteroids (long-term use)
- Diethylstilbestrol (exposure while in utero)
- Immunosuppressants used in organ transplantation
- Oral contraceptives (long-term use)

Causes of Abnormal Cervical Cytologic Findings

- Causes of ASC-US include atrophy, infection, inflammation, cervical dysplasia, and cervical cancer.
- Invasive cervical cancer is present in 0.1% to 0.2% of women with ASC-US and in 1% to 2% of women with high-grade squamous intraepithelial lesions (HSIL). About 5% to 10% of women with AGC have adenocarcinoma in situ or adenocarcinoma.

- About 5% of women with ASC-US, 24% to 94% of women with atypical squamous cells with high-grade intraepithelial lesion (ASC-H), 15% to 30% of women with low-grade squamous intraepithelial lesions (LSIL), 75% of women with HSIL, and up to 50% of women with AGC have moderate to severe cervical dysplasia.

Key Historical Features

✓ Gynecologic history

- History of sexually transmitted diseases
- Prior Pap smear abnormalities, positive results of HPV testing, abnormal findings in prior colposcopies, and treatment for abnormalities
- Frequency of prior Pap smears and date of last Pap smear
- Last normal menstrual period

✓ Sexual history

- Number of sexual partners
- Age at onset of sexual activity
- Sexual activity with partners at high risk of sexually transmitted diseases

✓ Obstetric history (early childbearing may increase the risk of cervical cancer)

✓ Associated symptoms

- Abnormal vaginal bleeding
- Postcoital bleeding
- Pelvic pain
- Vaginal discharge
- Foul vaginal odor
- Dyspareunia
- Dysuria
- Urinary frequency

✓ Menopausal status

✓ Medical history

- HIV infection
- Organ transplantation
- Lymphoproliferative disorders

✓ Medication use, especially oral contraceptives or immunosuppressants

✓ Social history
- Tobacco use
- Alcohol use
- Recreational drug use

Key Physical Findings

✓ External genital examination to evaluate for erythema (sign of infection with *Trichomonas* or *Candida* organisms) or ulcerative lesions, which may indicate herpes infection

✓ Speculum examination to evaluate for discharge, bleeding, or vaginal lesions (the vagina may appear erythematous with *Trichomonas* or *Candida* infection) and to evaluate the cervix for masses, erosions, ulcers, friability, or bleeding

✓ Bimanual examination to evaluate for any uterine or adnexal masses or tenderness

✓ Rectovaginal examination to evaluate for any masses or tenderness

Suggested Work-Up

The Bethesda 2001 classification system was used to create the American Society for Colposcopy and Cervical Pathology Consensus Guidelines in 2001 to distinguish women at risk for significant cervical disease from those with mild or no disease. The American College of Obstetrics and Gynecology also published guidelines for the management of abnormal Pap smears/cervical cytologic findings (Figs. 1-1 to 1-5). The guidelines involve substantial use of HPV DNA testing and colposcopy. Other testing used includes endocervical sampling, biopsy, and excisional procedures.

In pregnant women, endocervical sampling is not indicated and biopsies should be performed only for visible lesions that appear to be CIN grade 3, adenocarcinoma in situ, or cancer. In addition, excisional procedures should be considered in pregnant women only if a lesion discovered at colposcopy appears to be invasive cancer.

The following are recommendations for evaluation that are based upon cervical cytologic results. Algorithms are provided in Figures 1-1 to 1-5.

ASC-US   If HPV testing is positive, colposcopy should be performed with consideration of endocervical sampling with a brush or curette; if finding is negative, then the Pap smear should be repeated in 1 year

If HPV test result is negative, then a Pap smear should be repeated in 1 year; if HPV testing is not performed, other options include immediate colposcopy or repeat Pap smear at 6 and 12 months

If the patient is immunocompromised, then colposcopy should be performed immediately

In adolescents with ASC-US who are HPV positive, Pap smears may be repeated at 6 and 12 months or HPV testing may be undertaken at 12 months instead of immediate colposcopy, since clearance rate of HPV is high

ASC-H	Colposcopy should be performed with consideration of endocervical sampling
LSIL	Colposcopy should be performed with consideration of endocervical sampling
	In adolescents with LSIL, Pap smears may be repeated at 6 and 12 months or HPV testing may be repeated at 12 months instead of immediate colposcopy, since the clearance rate of HPV is high
HSIL	Colposcopy with endocervical sampling and biopsy should be performed. If the colposcopic finding is negative or inconclusive, then an excision should be performed
AGC	Colposcopy and endocervical sampling should be performed
	Endometrial sampling should be performed if the patient is older than 35 years or is at risk for endometrial cancer (abnormal bleeding, obesity, or oligomenorrhea)
	Figure 1-4 outlines the management of AGC based on initial cytology results.
AGC, favor neoplasia, or adenocarcinoma in situ	If the previously described work-up for AGC does not show invasive disease, then a diagnostic excisional procedure should be performed (cold-knife conization is preferred)

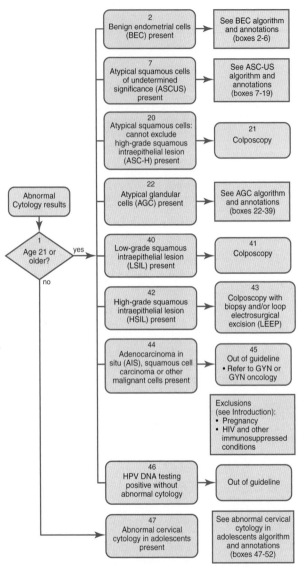

Figure 1-1. Initial management of abnormal cervical cytology (Pap smear) and human papillomavirus testing. Algorithm for initial abnormal cytologic result. Box numbers refer to algorithm boxes in Figure 1-1 to 1-5.

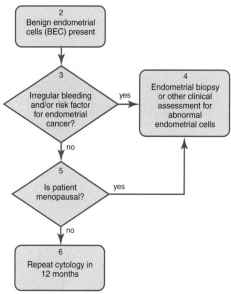

Figure 1-2. Initial management of abnormal cervical cytology (Pap smear) and human papillomavirus testing. Algorithm for benign endometrial cells (BEC).

Additional Work-Up

Test for HIV infection	In patients at risk
Chlamydia and gonorrhea cultures or a nucleic acid amplification test	In patients at risk
Urine pregnancy test	Should be performed before an invasive procedure if the patient may be pregnant
Wet mount evaluation	To evaluate for *Candida* infection, bacterial vaginosis, or *Trichomonas* infection if any of these conditions is suspected

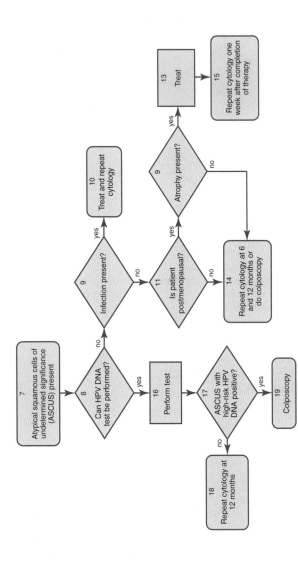

Figure I-3. Initial management of abnormal cervical cytology (Pap smear) and human papillomavirus testing. Algorithm for atypical squamous cells of undetermined significance (ASC-US).

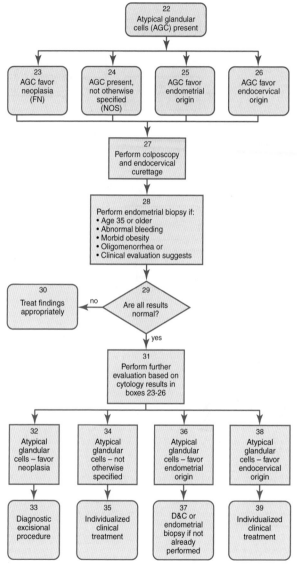

Figure 1-4. Initial management of abnormal cervical cytologic findings (Pap smear) and human papillomavirus testing. Algorithm for atypical glandular cells (AGC).

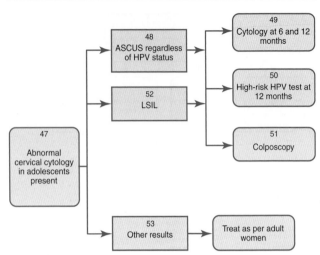

Figure 1-5. Initial management of abnormal cervical cytologic findings (Pap smear) and human papillomavirus testing. Algorithm for abnormal cervical cytologic findings in adolescents (younger than 21 years).

FURTHER READING

American College of Obstetrics and Gynecology: ACOG Practice Bulletin number 66, September 2005. Management of abnormal cervical cytology and histology. Obstet Gynecol 2005;106:645-664.

Apgar BS, Brotzman G: Management of cervical cytologic abnormalities. Am Fam Physician 2004;70:1905-1916.

Apgar BS, Zoschnick L, Wright TC Jr: The 2001 Bethesda system terminology. Am Fam Physician 2003;68:1992-1998.

Buechler EJ: Pap tests and HPV infection. Postgrad Med 2005;118(2):37-46.

Bundrick JB, Cook DA, Gostout BS: Screening for cervical cancer and initial treatment of patients with abnormal results from Papanicolaou testing. Mayo Clin Proc 2005;80: 1063-1108.

Institute for Clinical Systems Improvement. Initial Management of Abnormal Cervical Cytology (Pap Smear) and HPV Testing. Bloomington, MN: Institute for Clinical Systems Improvement, 2006.

Solomon D, Davey D, Kurman R, et al: The 2001 Bethesda System: terminology for reporting results of cervical cytology. Forum Group Members; Bethesda 2001 Workshop. JAMA 2002;287:2114-2119.

U.S. Preventive Services Task Force: Screening for Cervical Cancer. Available at http://www.ahrq.gov. Accessed on Web 8/8/07.

ABNORMAL PREMENOPAUSAL UTERINE BLEEDING

Theodore O'Connell

In women of childbearing age, abnormal uterine bleeding includes any change in menstrual period frequency, duration, or amount of flow, as well as bleeding between cycles. A menstrual cycle of fewer than 21 days or more than 35 days is considered abnormal. Likewise, a menstrual flow of fewer than 2 days or more than 7 days is abnormal.

When abnormal uterine bleeding is evaluated (Figs. 2-1 and 2-2), it is important to make certain that the bleeding is not from a gastrointestinal or urinary source. Once it is clear that the bleeding is vaginal, pregnancy should be the first consideration in women of childbearing age. After pregnancy has been ruled out, iatrogenic causes of abnormal uterine bleeding should be considered. Medications linked to abnormal premenopausal uterine bleeding are outlined later in this chapter. After pregnancy and iatrogenic causes have been excluded, systemic conditions should be considered. These systemic causes and the suggested workup, outlined later in the chapter, include thyroid, hematologic, pituitary, hepatic, adrenal, and hypothalamic disorders.

Genital tract disease should be considered. Diagnoses that should be considered include cervical pathologic processes, sexually transmitted disease, trauma, uterine fibroids, endometrial polyps, endometrial hyperplasia and atypia, and endometrial cancer.

Dysfunctional uterine bleeding occurs during the childbearing years, but the diagnosis is one of exclusion that should be made only after pregnancy, iatrogenic causes, systemic conditions, and obvious genital tract disease have been ruled out.

Further evaluation of abnormal uterine bleeding depends on the patient's age and the presence of risk factors for endometrial cancer. These risk factors include anovulatory cycles, obesity, nulliparity, age greater than 35 years, and tamoxifen therapy. Anovulation occurs at the extremes of reproductive age (during the postmenarchal and perimenopausal periods).

Because endometrial cancer is rare in 15- to 18-year-old girls, dysfunctional uterine bleeding in most adolescents can be treated safely with hormone therapy and observation, without the need for diagnostic testing.

Of cases of endometrial carcinoma, 20% to 25% occur before menopause, and the risk of developing endometrial cancer increases with age. Thus, the American College of Obstetricians and Gynecologists recommends endometrial evaluation in women aged 35 and older who have abnormal uterine bleeding. Endometrial evaluation is also recommended for patients younger than 35 who are at high risk for endometrial cancer. Women with vaginal bleeding who are younger than 35 years and have no identifiable risk factors for neoplasia can be assumed to have dysfunctional bleeding and treated accordingly. However, if bleeding continues in a patient at low risk for neoplasia despite medical management, endometrial evaluation is indicated.

Endometrial evaluation may be accomplished by endometrial biopsy, transvaginal ultrasonography, saline-infusion sonohysterography, dilatation and curettage, or hysteroscopy with biopsy. Endometrial evaluation usually proceeds with endometrial biopsy, which can be performed in the office using the Pipelle technique. The efficacy of transvaginal ultrasonography in the premenopausal population is not as well defined as it is in postmenopausal women. For this reason, endometrial evaluation usually begins with endometrial biopsy. However, because endometrial biopsy may miss a significant percentage of benign endometrial lesions such as polyps and fibroids, some clinicians recommend proceeding to saline-infusion sonohysterography or dilatation and curettage with hysteroscopy.

Medications Linked to Abnormal Premenopausal Uterine Bleeding

Anticoagulants

Antipsychotics

Corticosteroids

Herbal and other supplements

Hormonal contraception

Intrauterine devices

Selective serotonin reuptake inhibitors

Tamoxifen

Thyroid hormone replacement

Causes of Abnormal Premenopausal Uterine Bleeding

Adenomyosis

Adrenal hyperplasia and Cushing disease

Atrophic endometrium

Bleeding disorders

Cervical carcinoma

Cervical dysplasia

Cervical polyp

Cervicitis

Dysfunctional uterine bleeding

Endometrial carcinoma

Endometrial hyperplasia

Endometrial polyp

Endometritis

Estrogen-producing ovarian tumors

Hyperprolactinemia

Hypothalamic suppression (stress, weight loss, excessive exercise)

Hyperthyroidism

Hypothyroidism

Leiomyomata

Leiomyosarcoma

Leukemia

Liver failure

Medications and herbal supplements

Myometritis

Pituitary adenoma

Polycystic ovary syndrome

Pregnancy (intrauterine or ectopic)

Pregnancy-related conditions

- Abruptio placentae
- Ectopic pregnancy
- Miscarriage
- Placenta previa
- Trophoblastic disease

Renal disease

Salpingitis

Testosterone-producing ovarian tumors

Thrombocytopenia

Trauma (foreign body, abrasions, lacerations, sexual abuse or assault)

Key Historical Features

✓ Frequency, duration, and severity of flow

✓ Normal cycle pattern

✓ Method of contraception

✓ Compliance with hormonal contraception if it is being used

✓ Sexual activity

✓ Postcoital bleeding

✓ Pelvic pain

✓ Easy bruising or tendency to bleed

✓ Jaundice or history of hepatitis

✓ Stress

✓ Excessive exercise

✓ Medical history

✓ Surgical history

✓ Obstetric and gynecologic history

✓ Medications

✓ Systemic symptoms

- Fatigue
- Nausea or vomiting
- Weight gain or weight loss
- Heat or cold intolerance
- Constipation
- Sweating
- Palpitations
- Urinary frequency
- Easy bruising
- Jaundice
- Hirsutism
- Acne
- Headache
- Galactorrhea
- Visual field disturbance

Key Physical Findings

✓ Assessment of vital signs

✓ General assessment of health and evaluation for obesity

✓ Search for evidence of eating disorders

✓ Thyroid examination for thyromegaly or thyroid tenderness

✓ Cardiovascular examination for tachycardia

✓ Skin examination for acne or acanthosis nigricans (signs of polycystic ovary syndrome or diabetes mellitus); also evaluation for bruising as a sign of coagulopathy and for jaundice

✓ Breast examination for galactorrhea

✓ Pelvic examination to evaluate for vulvar or vaginal lesions, signs of trauma, cervical polyps or dysplasia, cervical motion tenderness, uterine enlargement, uterine tenderness, or adnexal masses

✓ Extremity examination for edema

Suggested Work-Up

Pregnancy test	To evaluate for pregnancy
Pap smear	To evaluate for cervical dysplasia
Cultures for gonorrhea and chlamydia or nucleic acid amplification tests	If infection is suspected or the patient is at risk for sexually transmitted disease
Complete blood cell count (CBC)	If bleeding is heavy or prolonged and anemia is suspected
Endometrial biopsy *or* transvaginal ultrasonography *or* saline infusion sonohysterography *or* dilatation and curettage with hysteroscopy	Recommended in women aged 35 and older with abnormal uterine bleeding; also recommended for patients younger than 35 who are at high risk for endometrial cancer and for patients at low risk who continue bleeding abnormally despite medical management. See previous text for an explanation of benefits and drawbacks of each.

Additional Work-Up

Transvaginal ultrasonography	If there is uterine enlargement or an adnexal mass
Thyroid-stimulating hormone (TSH) measurement	If hypothyroidism or hyperthyroidism is suspected
Prolactin level measurement	If pituitary adenoma or hyperprolactinemia is suspected

Blood glucose measurement	If diabetes mellitus is suspected
Liver function tests and prothrombin time measurement	If liver disease is suspected
CBC with measurements of platelet count, prothrombin time, and partial thromboplastin time	If coagulopathy is suspected
Dehydroepiandrosterone sulfate (DHEAS), free testosterone, and 17α-hydroxyprogesterone measurements	If ovarian or adrenal tumor is suspected on the basis of signs of hyperandrogenism
von Willebrand factor measurement	If von Willebrand disease is suspected
Blood urea nitrogen (BUN), creatinine, and TSH measurements	If edema is present
Colposcopy	If cervical dysplasia is found on Pap smear

FURTHER READING

ACOG Community on Practice Bulletins—American College of Obstetrics and Gynecology: ACOG practice bulletin: management of anovulatory bleeding. Int J Gynaecol Obstet 2001;73:263-271.

Albers JR, Hull SH, Wesley RM: Abnormal uterine bleeding. Am Fam Physician 2004;69:1915-1926.

Apgar BS: Dysmenorrhea and dysfunctional uterine bleeding. Prim Care 1997;24:161-178.

Chen BH, Giudice LC: Dysfunctional uterine bleeding. West J Med 1998;169:280-284.

Davidson KG, Dubinsky TJ: Ultrasonographic evaluation of the endometrium in postmenopausal vaginal bleeding. Radiol Clin North Am 2003;41:769-780.

Elford KJ, Spence JE: The forgotten female: pediatric and adolescent gynecological concerns and their reproductive consequences. J Pediatr Adolesc Gynecol 2002;15:65-77.

Goldstein SR: Abnormal uterine bleeding: the role of ultrasound. Radiol Clin North Am 2005;44:901-910.

Goldstein SR, Zeltser I, Horan CK, et al: Ultrasonography-based triage for perimenopausal patients with abnormal uterine bleeding. Am J Obstet Gynecol 1997;177:102-108.

Goodman A: Abnormal genital tract bleeding. Clin Cornerstone 2000;3(1):25-35.

Kilbourn C, Richards C: Abnormal uterine bleeding. Postgrad Med 2001;109:137-140.

Schrager S: Abnormal uterine bleeding associated with hormonal contraception. Am Fam Physician 2002;65:2073-2080.

Smith-Bindman R, Kerlikowske K, Feldstein VA, et al: Endovaginal ultrasound to exclude endometrial cancer and other endometrial abnormalities. JAMA 1998;280:1510-1517.

Tabor A, Watt HC, Wald NJ: Endometrial thickness as a test for endometrial cancer in women with postmenopausal vaginal bleeding. Obstet Gynecol 2002;99:663-670.

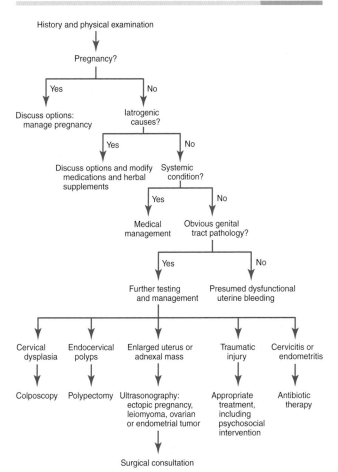

Figure 2-1. Abnormal uterine bleeding in women of childbearing age. Sequential steps through the differential diagnosis of abnormal uterine bleeding in women of childbearing age.

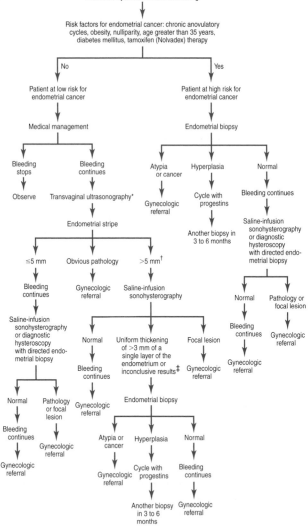

Figure 2-2. Presumed dysfunctional uterine bleeding in women of childbearing age: evaluation based on risk factors for endometrial cancer.

---

*Transvaginal ultrasonography ideally is performed during the late proliferative stage.
†Some investigators consider an endometrial stripe of 7 to 8 mm or larger to be abnormal in premenopausal or perimenopausal women.
‡These determinants are based on information from Goldstein SR, Zeltser I, Horan CK, Snyder JR, Schwartz LB. Ultrasonography-based triage for perimenopausal patients with abnormal uterine bleeding. Am J Obstet Gynecol 1997;177:102-108.

3 ADNEXAL MASS

Kathleen Dor

The key element in the evaluation of an adnexal mass is whether the mass is malignant or benign. Not only can an adnexal mass represent ovarian cancer but it can also be metastatic disease from the breast or gastrointestinal tract or other gynecological neoplasms. Of all ovarian masses, 45% in postmenopausal women are cancer, in comparison with 13% in premenopausal women

Most cases of ovarian cancer are diagnosed at an advanced stage, at which point the overall 5-year survival rate is 30% to 55%. However, in women in whom stage I ovarian cancer is diagnosed, the 5-year survival rate is greater than 90%. Risk factors for the development of ovarian cancer include postmenopausal status, a family history of breast or ovarian cancer, nulliparity, infertility, and endometriosis. Other than prophylactic oophorectomy, the only method of decreasing the risk of ovarian cancer is taking combined oral contraceptives.

Causes of an Adnexal Mass

Gynecologic Causes

Benign

- Ectopic pregnancy
- Endometrioma
- Functional cyst
- Hydrosalpinx
- Leiomyomata
- Mature teratoma
- Mucinous cystadenoma
- Polycystic ovarian syndrome
- Serous cystadenoma
- Tubo-ovarian abscess

Malignant

- Epithelial cell ovarian carcinoma
- Fallopian tube carcinoma
- Germ cell tumor
- Gonadal stromal tumor
- Malignant mesodermal sarcoma

- Metastatic breast cancer
- Metastatic uterine cancer
- Ovarian lymphoma

Nongynecologic Causes

Benign

- Appendiceal abscess or mucocele
- Bladder distension
- Bladder diverticulum
- Diverticular abscess
- Hematoma
- Hernia
- Nerve sheath tumors
- Paratubal cyst
- Pelvic kidney
- Ureteral diverticulum

Malignant

- Gastrointestinal cancers
- Retroperitoneal sarcomas

Key Historical Features

✓ General features

- Unintentional weight loss and decreased energy, which may indicate cancer
- Fevers, which may indicate an infectious process
- Associated obesity, hirsutism, and acne, which may occur with polycystic ovarian syndrome

✓ Gynecologic features

- Most recent normal menstrual period
- Contraception use
- Sexual history
- Menopausal status
- Date and results of last mammogram
- Breast lumps or skin changes
- Associated pain (acute pain may occur with ovarian torsion, cyst rupture, ectopic pregnancy, appendicitis; gradually worsening pain suggests cancer; chronic pain may occur with a tubo-ovarian abscess; cyclic pain may represent endometriosis)
- Obstetric history, including prior ectopic pregnancies

- History of sexually transmitted diseases, pelvic inflammatory disease (which increases the risk for ectopic pregnancy), hydrosalpinx, or tubo-ovarian abscess
- Associated symptoms, such as vaginal bleeding (ectopic pregnancy, uterine cancer, estrogen-producing ovarian tumor), vaginal discharge (pelvic inflammatory disease), increased urinary frequency (ovarian neoplasm), or abdominal distension (ovarian neoplasm)

✓ Gastrointestinal features

- Rectal bleeding and change in bowel habits, which may indicate colon cancer
- Date and results of last appropriate colon cancer screening
- History of colon polyps

✓ Family history, especially of ovarian, breast, and colon cancer

Key Physical Findings

✓ Dermatologic examination

- Hirsutism, which may indicate virilization caused by a testosterone-producing tumor

✓ Gynecologic examination

- Clitoromegaly (part of virilization; detected through evaluation of the external genitalia)
- Any cervical or vaginal lesions or evidence of infection (detected through speculum examination)
- Malignant mass (often firm, immobile and irregular; detected through bimanual examination to evaluate the size, mobility, firmness, regularity, and tenderness of the mass)

✓ Breast examination for any evidence of malignancy

✓ Gastrointestinal examination

- Masses, tenderness, or organomegaly (detected through abdominal examination)
- Rectal masses or occult bleeding (detected through rectal examination)

Suggested Work-Up

Urine pregnancy test	To evaluate for pregnancy in a woman of childbearing age
Transvaginal ultrasonography	According to the latest guidelines from the American College of Obstetricians and

	Gynecologists (ACOG), transvaginal ultrasonography is the first choice of imaging in asymptomatic women with a pelvic mass
Cancer antigen 125 (CA 125) measurement	Of women with epithelial ovarian cancer, 80% have an elevated CA 125 level; however, it is elevated in only 50% of women with stage 1 disease, and its measurement is therefore not a good screening test
	In addition, CA 125 level is rarely elevated with germ cell, stromal, or mucinous ovarian cancers
	The sensitivity and specificity of CA 125 in diagnosing malignant adnexal masses is highest after menopause
	Elevation of CA 125 level in a postmenopausal woman with an adnexal mass is very suggestive of cancer
Complete blood cell count (CBC)	To evaluate for anemia or infection

Additional Work-Up

Quantitative β–human chorionic gonadotropin (β-hCG) measurement	To evaluate for malignant germ cell tumors, especially in premenopausal women
α-Fetoprotein measurement	If malignant germ cell tumor is suspected
Lactate dehydrogenase (LDH) measurement	If malignant germ cell tumor is suspected
Inhibin A and inhibin B measurement	If ovarian granulosa cell tumor is suspected
Gonorrhea and chlamydia nucleic acid amplification tests or culture	To evaluate for gonorrhea and *Chlamydia* infections if suspected or if patient is at risk
Pap smear	If cervical cancer screening is due
Colonoscopy	If colon cancer is suspected or if colon cancer screening is due

Upper gastrointestinal endoscopy	If gastric cancer is suspected
Fecal occult blood testing	To evaluate for risk of colon or other gastrointestinal cancers
Mammography	If breast cancer is suspected or if breast cancer screening is due
Computed tomographic scan of abdomen and pelvis (with contrast media)	To evaluate for metastases or an unknown primary cancer
Endometrial biopsy	To evaluate for uterine cancer if postmenopausal uterine bleeding is present or a thickened endometrial lining is visible on ultrasonography
Magnetic resonance imaging (MRI) of pelvis	To evaluate pelvic masses whose ultrasound findings are indeterminate

FURTHER READING

American College of Obstetricians and Gynecologists: ACOG Practice Bulletin. Management of adnexal masses. Obstet Gynecol 2007;110:201-214.

Gostout BS, Brewer MA: Guidelines for referral of the patient with an adnexal mass. Clin Obstet Gynecol 2006;49:448-458.

McDonald JM, Modesitt SC: The incidental postmenopausal adnexal mass. Clin Obstet Gynecol 2006;49:506-516.

Russell DJ: The female pelvic mass: diagnosis and management. Med Clin North Am 1995;79:1481-1493.

Theodore O'Connell

Primary amenorrhea is defined as the absence of menses by 16 years of age in the presence of normal growth and secondary sexual characteristics or lack of menses by 14 years of age in the absence of secondary sexual characteristics. In the classification of primary amenorrhea, *hypogonadism* refers to gonads that are not functioning, and this condition is associated with a hypoestrogenic state; *eugonadism* refers to gonads that maintain normal steroidogenesis, and this condition is associated with a well-estrogenized state. An evaluation of breast development can be used to determine a patient's estrogen status. The pelvic examination then further narrows the potential causes by determining the presence or absence of a normal mullerian system.

The most common cause of primary amenorrhea is primary ovarian failure resulting from gonadal dysgenesis, most commonly as a result of Turner syndrome. The second most common cause of primary amenorrhea is congenital absence of the uterus and vagina, followed by idiopathic hypogonadotropic hypogonadism. Another cause of secondary amenorrhea involves eating disorder. The incidences of eating disorders such as anorexia and bulimia are highest during the adolescent years. Anorexia nervosa has a prevalence of 1% in the United States. The so-called female athlete triad—characterized by disordered eating, osteoporosis or osteopenia, and amenorrhea in the setting of excessive exercise—overlaps with eating disorders.

The first step in the evaluation of primary amenorrhea (Fig. 4-1) is documentation of the history and a physical examination. If secondary sexual characteristics are not present, follicle-stimulating hormone (FSH) and luteinizing hormone (LH) levels should be measured. FSH and LH levels lower than 5 IU/L indicate hypogonadotropic hypogonadism. If the FSH level exceeds 20 IU/L and the LH level exceeds 40 IU/L, hypergonadotropic hypogonadism is present; in that case, karyotype analysis is indicated.

If secondary sexual characteristics are present, ultrasonography of the uterus should be performed. If the uterus is absent or abnormal, karyotype analysis is indicated. If the uterus is present and normal, the patient should be examined for evidence of an outflow obstruction.

Medications Linked to Amenorrhea

Butyrophenones

Contraceptive medications

Divalproex

Domperidone

Haloperidol

H_2 blockers

Methyldopa

Metoclopramide

Opiates

Phenothiazine

Psychotropic medications

Reserpine

Risperidone

Sulpiride

Verapamil

Causes of Primary Amenorrhea

Eugonadism

Androgen insensitivity

Cervical atresia

Congenital absence of the uterus and vagina

Imperforate hymen

Polycystic ovarian syndrome

Transverse vaginal septum

17-Ketoreductase deficiency

Hypergonadotropic Hypogonadism

Ovarian failure (caused by chromosomal abnormality, previous irradiation, or previous chemotherapy)

Pseudo-ovarian failure

Turner syndrome

46, XX Gonadal dysgenesis

46, XY Gonadal dysgenesis

Hypogonadotropic Hypogonadism

Congenital adrenal hyperplasia

Congenital central nervous system (CNS) defects

Constitutional delay

Craniopharyngioma

Cushing syndrome

Diabetes (poorly controlled)

Eating disorders (anorexia nervosa and bulimia nervosa)

Hyperprolactinemia

Hypopituitarism

Hypothyroidism

Idiopathic hypogonadotropic hypogonadism

Isolated gonadotropin-releasing hormone (GnRH)
deficiency

Juvenile rheumatoid arthritis

Malabsorptive bowel disease

Malignant tumor

Marijuana use

Pituitary adenoma (prolactinoma)

Pseudohypoparathyroidism

Psychological stress

Systemic disorders

Key Historical Features

✓   Menarche and menstrual history

✓   Sexual history

✓   Diet history

✓   Physical activity

✓   Medical history, including history of chemotherapy
    or irradiation

✓   Surgical history

✓   Medications

✓   Family history, especially of infertility, genetic defects, and menstrual
    disorders

✓   Symptoms of hyperthyroidism or hypothyroidism

✓   Acne or hirsutism

✓   Headache or visual disturbances

✓   Anosmia or galactorrhea

✓   Cyclic abdominal pain

✓   Breast changes

✓   Easy bruising

Key Physical Findings

✓ Vital signs

✓ Height and weight compared against normative data

✓ Body mass index

✓ Breast development

✓ Pubertal development according to Tanner staging

✓ Signs of an eating disorder, such as parotid gland enlargement, Russell's sign, or dental erosions

✓ Thyroid examination

✓ Abdominal examination for masses

✓ Pelvic examination for imperforate hymen, transverse vaginal septum, clitoral hypertrophy, or undescended testes

✓ Rectal examination for skin tags, fissures, or occult blood that may indicate inflammatory bowel disease

✓ Evaluation for striae, buffalo hump, central obesity, or proximal muscle weakness

Suggested Work-Up

Pregnancy test	To rule out pregnancy
Serum FSH and LH measurement	Should be undertaken if secondary sexual characteristics are not present
	FSH level higher than 30 and up to 40 IU/L is suggestive of premature ovarian failure; LH level is more suppressed than FSH level when amenorrhea is caused by suppression of the hypothalamic-pituitary-ovarian axis
Prolactin level measurement	To evaluate for hyperprolactinemia
Ultrasonography of the uterus	Should be performed if primary amenorrhea is present and secondary sexual characteristics are also present
	If the uterus is absent or abnormal, karyotype analysis should be performed; if the uterus is present and normal, the patient should be

evaluated for evidence of outflow obstruction

Additional Work-Up

Karyotype analysis	If FSH level is persistently elevated, karyotype analysis is necessary to evaluate for a chromosomal abnormality
Complete blood cell count (CBC), erythrocyte sedimentation rate (ESR) measurement, thyroid-stimulating hormone (TSH) measurement, liver function tests, electrolyte measurements, blood urea nitrogen (BUN) measurement, creatinine measurement, blood glucose measurement, and urinalysis	If pubertal delay is present or systemic illness is suspected
Serum estradiol measurement	To confirm hypoestrogenism if premature ovarian failure is suspected
Serum testosterone and dehydroepiandrosterone sulfate (DHEAS) measurement	To evaluate for hyperandrogenism if signs of androgen excess are present
Magnetic resonance imaging (MRI) of the sella turcica	If pituitary tumor is suspected (prolactin level > 100 ng/mL)
Radiography of the hand and wrist	If short stature is present, to clarify skeletal maturation for chronologic age

FURTHER READING

Adams-Hillard PJ, Deitch HR: Menstrual disorders in the college age female. Pediatr Clin North Am 2005;52:179-197.

Kazis K, Iglesias E: The female athlete triad. Adolesc Med 2003;14:87-95.

Master-Hunter T, Heiman DL: Amenorrhea: evaluation and treatment. Am Fam Physician 2006;73:1374-1382.

Pletcher JR, Slap GB: Menstrual disorders: amenorrhea. Pediatr Clin North Am 1999;46:505-518.

Timmreck LS, Reindollar RH: Contemporary issues in primary amenorrhea. Obstet Gynecol Clin 2003;30:287-302.

Warren MP: Evaluation of secondary amenorrhea. J Clin Endocrinol Metab 1996;81:437-442.

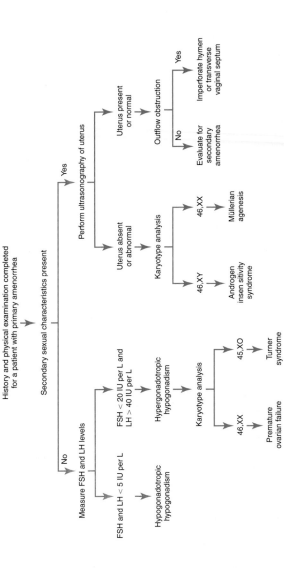

Figure 4-1. Evaluation of primary amenorrhea. *(From Master-Hunter T, Heiman DL: Amenorrhea: evaluation and treatment. Am Fam Physician 2006; 73:1374-1382.)*

5 AMENORRHEA: SECONDARY

Theodore O'Connell

Secondary amenorrhea is the absence of menses for 3 months in women with previously normal menstruation or for 9 months in women with previous oligomenorrhea. Secondary amenorrhea is more common than primary amenorrhea. The most common cause of secondary amenorrhea is pregnancy. Thyroid disease and hyperprolactinemia are also common causes of secondary amenorrhea.

Once pregnancy, thyroid disease, and hyperprolactinemia are ruled out as potential causes (Fig. 5-1), the remaining causes of secondary amenorrhea are classified as eugonadotropic amenorrhea, hypogonadotropic hypogonadism, and hypergonadotropic hypogonadism. Outflow tract obstruction and hyperandrogenic chronic anovulation are two common causes of eugonadotropic amenorrhea. Polycystic ovary syndrome is the most common cause of hyperandrogenic chronic anovulation.

Clinically, it is helpful to distinguish patients who have secondary amenorrhea as those with and those without hirsutism or signs of androgen excess. This can be done by history documentation and physical examination, as well as by laboratory studies. Physical examination may reveal hirsutism, acanthosis nigricans, acne, or clitoromegaly.

Medications Linked to Amenorrhea

Butyrophenones

Contraceptive medications

Divalproex

Domperidone

Haloperidol

H_2 blockers

Methyldopa

Metoclopramide

Opiates

Phenothiazine

Psychotropic medications

Reserpine

Risperidone

Sulpiride

Verapamil

Causes of Secondary Amenorrhea

Eugonadism

Acromegaly

Androgen-secreting tumor

Asherman syndrome

Cervical stenosis

Congenital adrenal hyperplasia

Cushing disease

Exogenous androgens (anabolic steroids)

Hyperprolactinemia

Ovarian stromal hypertrophy

Polycystic ovary syndrome

Pregnancy

Thyroid disease

Hypergonadotropic Hypogonadism

Postmenopausal ovarian failure

Premature ovarian failure

Hypogonadotropic Hypogonadism

Anorexia nervosa

Bulimia nervosa

Celiac disease

Central nervous system (CNS) tumor

Chronic liver disease

Chronic renal insufficiency

Cranial irradiation

Cystic fibrosis

Depression

Diabetes mellitus

Excessive exercise

Human immunodeficiency virus (HIV) infection

Immunodeficiency

Inflammatory bowel disease

Marijuana use

Psychologic stress

Renal disease

Sickle cell disease

Thalassemia major

Thyroid disease

Key Historical Features

✓ Menarche and menstrual history

✓ Sexual history

✓ Diet history

✓ Physical activity

✓ Medical history, including history of chemotherapy or irradiation

✓ Surgical history

✓ Medications

✓ Family history, especially of infertility, genetic defects, and menstrual disorders

✓ Symptoms of hyperthyroidism or hypothyroidism

✓ Acne or hirsutism

✓ Headache or visual disturbances

✓ Anosmia or galactorrhea

✓ Cyclic abdominal pain

✓ Breast changes

✓ Easy bruising

Key Physical Findings

✓ Vital signs

✓ Height and weight compared against normative data

✓ Body mass index

✓ Breast development

✓ Pubertal development according to Tanner staging

✓ Signs of an eating disorder, such as parotid gland enlargement, Russell's sign, or dental erosions

✓ Thyroid examination

✓ Abdominal examination for masses

✓ Pelvic examination for imperforate hymen, transverse vaginal septum, clitoral hypertrophy, or undescended testes

✓   Rectal examination for skin tags, fissures, or occult blood that may indicate inflammatory bowel disease

✓   Evaluation for striae, buffalo hump, central obesity, or proximal muscle weakness

Suggested Work-Up

Pregnancy test	To evaluate for pregnancy
Prolactin level measurement	To evaluate for hyperprolactinemia
Thyroid-stimulating hormone (TSH) measurement	To evaluate for subclinical hypothyroidism
Luteinizing hormone (LH) and follicle-stimulating hormone (FSH) measurement	If polycystic ovarian syndrome is suspected (LH/FSH ratio may be elevated)

Additional Work-Up

Progestogen challenge test	If prolactin and TSH levels are normal, progestogen challenge is used to help evaluate for a patent outflow tract
	A negative progestogen challenge test result indicates an outflow tract abnormality or inadequate estrogenization
Estrogen/progestogen challenge test	Used to differentiate abnormal outflow tract from inadequate estrogenization; a negative finding usually indicates an outflow tract obstruction, and a positive finding indicates an abnormality within the hypothalamic-pituitary-ovarian axis
Testosterone and dehydroepiandrosterone sulfate (DHEAS) measurements	If signs of androgen excess are present, these evaluations are for adrenal disease and androgen-secreting ovarian tumors
Estradiol level	To confirm hypoestrogenism if premature ovarian failure is suspected

17-Hydroxyprogesterone measurement before and after ACTH injection	If adult-onset congenital adrenal hyperplasia is suspected
Measurement of urinary free cortisol and serum electrolytes	If Addison disease is suspected clinically in the setting of premature ovarian failure
Magnetic resonance imaging (MRI) of the sella turcica	To evaluate for pituitary tumor if the prolactin level exceeds 100 ng/mL
Hysterosalpingography, hysteroscopy, or sonohysterography	If Asherman syndrome is suspected in the setting of outflow tract obstruction

FURTHER READING

Adams Hillard PJ, Deitch HR: Menstrual disorders in the college age female. Pediatr Clin North Am 2005;52:179-197.

Kazis K, Iglesias E: The female athlete triad. Adolesc Med 2003;14:87-95.

Kiningham RB, Apgar BS, Schwenk TL: Evaluation of amenorrhea. Am Fam Physician 1996;53:1185-1194.

Master-Hunter T, Heiman DL: Amenorrhea: evaluation and treatment. Am Fam Physician 2006;73:1374-1382.

Pickett CA: Diagnosis and management of pituitary tumors: recent advances. Primary Care 2003;30:765-789.

Pletcher JR, Slap GB: Menstrual disorders: amenorrhea. Pediatr Clin North Am 1999;46:505-518.

Speroff L, Fritz MA: Amenorrhea. In: Clinical Gynecologic Endocrinology and Infertility, 7th ed. Philadelphia: Lippincott Williams & Wilkins, 2005:401-464.

Warren MP: Evaluation of secondary amenorrhea. J Clin Endocrinol Metab 1996;81:437-442.

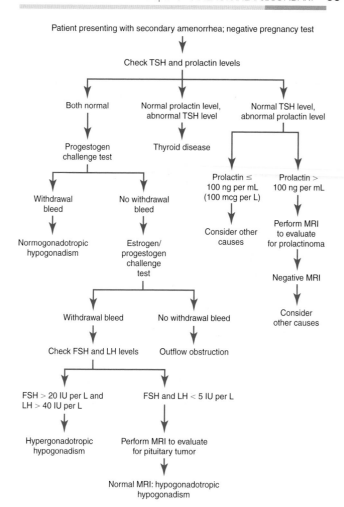

Figure 5-1. Evaluation of secondary amenorrhea. *(From Master-Hunter T, Heiman DL: Amenorrhea: evaluation and treatment. Am Fam Physician 2006;73:1374-1382.)*

6 PALPABLE BREAST MASS

Teri Kim and Theodore O'Connell

Approximately 190,000 new cases of breast cancer are diagnosed annually in the United States; however, most breast masses are benign. In order to diagnose these cancers, well over 1 million breast biopsies are performed each year. Fibroadenoma is the most common benign breast mass, whereas invasive ductal carcinoma is the most common malignancy.

After the patient history is obtained, a clinical breast examination is performed. Benign masses generally are smooth, soft to firm, and mobile, with well-defined margins and no skin changes. Malignant masses generally are hard, immobile, and fixed to surrounding skin and soft tissue, with poorly defined or irregular margins. With infections such as cellulitis and mastitis, the masses usually are erythematous, tender, and warm to the touch. However, similar symptoms may occur in patients with inflammatory breast cancer.

After the clinical breast examination, the initial step in the evaluation of a palpable dominant breast mass is to determine whether it is cystic or solid. This distinction may be made by targeted ultrasonography and diagnostic mammography or by fine-needle aspiration (FNA).

The next step in evaluating a patient with a palpable breast mass is determined by the patient's age and the physician's experience with performing office-based FNA. FNA of a palpable lesion is often a better choice than image-guided biopsy because it is easier on the patient, and aspiration directed to the palpable lesion will confirm the presence of the tumor at the site and obviate the need for image guidance at the time of surgical excision. FNA is preferable to core biopsy for small lesions because it is easier and more accurate for guiding a small-gauge needle into the lesion. Large masses can be diagnosed through either FNA or core biopsy.

FNA is used to aspirate cystic fluid or sample solid lesions for cytologic study. If FNA reveals fluid that is clear yellow, straw-colored, green, or brown (typical features of benign cystic fluid), the fluid can be discarded. The dominant mass should disappear, and a clinical breast examination should be repeated in 4 to 6 weeks. If there is residual mass after cyst aspiration or if the fluid is bloody, the evaluation proceeds with mammography, targeted ultrasonography, or core-needle biopsy. If FNA reveals a solid lesion, the evaluation proceeds with diagnostic mammography. Ultrasonography may be considered in women younger than 40 years.

If FNA is not possible during the initial presentation, ultrasonography should be considered to rule out cystic disease and delineate lesion margins.

The goal of biopsy is to direct a therapeutic course. Minimally invasive techniques are preferable to open surgical biopsy because they avoid both scarring and additional procedures that may not be necessary. If the lesion is cancerous, the goal is to establish a diagnosis as quickly and nontraumatically as possible in order to facilitate a discussion about treatment options.

Women presenting with a breast mass must undergo bilateral diagnostic mammography. Diagnostic mammography can be performed in women at any age; however, in women younger than 40 years, ultrasonography directed at the area of concern is the preferred study because the density of glandular breast tissue lowers the sensitivity of mammography.

The triple test is the combination of clinical breast examination, imaging, and tissue sampling. When the three assessments are performed adequately and produce concordant results, the diagnostic accuracy of the triple test approaches 100%. Discordant results or results that cannot be evaluated may indicate the need for excisional biopsy. The triple test score (TTS) was developed to help physicians interpret discordant results. A 3-point scale is used to score each component of the triple test (1 = benign, 2 = suspicious, and 3 = malignant). A TTS of 3 or 4 is consistent with a benign lesion. A TTS of 6 or more indicates possible malignancy that may necessitate surgical intervention. In patients with a TTS of 5, excisional biopsy is recommended for obtaining a definitive diagnosis. If all three elements indicate benign disease, the patient may be monitored with another examination in 4 to 6 weeks.

Causes of Breast Masses

Abscess

Atypical hyperplasia of the breast

Benign cyst

Carcinoma

- Ductal invasive carcinoma
- Inflammatory carcinoma
- Intraductal carcinoma in situ
- Lobular carcinoma in situ
- Lobular invasive carcinoma
- Medullary invasive carcinoma
- Paget disease

Cellulitis

Fat necrosis

Fibroadenoma

Fibrocystic change

Lipoma

Mammary duct ectasia

Mastitis

Papilloma

Phyllodes tumor

Risk Factors for Breast Cancer

Advancing age

Female sex

Personal history of breast cancer

History of benign breast disease, especially cystic disease, proliferative types of hyperplasia, and atypical hyperplasia

Family history of breast cancer in a first-degree relative or several second-degree relatives, especially if the cancer was diagnosed premenopausally

Early menarche

Late menopause

First childbirth after age 30

Nulliparity

Not breastfeeding

BRCA1 and *BRCA2* gene mutations

Obesity

Previous breast lesions

Radiation exposure

Oral contraceptive use (may minimally increase risk)

Estrogen replacement therapy (possibly increases risk)

Alcohol consumption

White race

High social economic status

Key Historical Features

✓   Exact location of mass

✓   Duration of mass

✓   Changes in size over time

✓   Change in relation to menstrual cycle

✓   Pain

✓   Fever, swelling, or redness

✓   Nipple discharge

✓   Medical history, especially of the following:

- History of breast or ovarian cancer
- Previous breast masses and biopsies
- Recent breast trauma
- Radiation therapy or chemotherapy
- Any radiation exposure

✓   Surgical history

✓   Obstetric and gynecologic history

- Age at menarche
- Age at first childbearing
- Number of pregnancies and number of children
- Age at menopause
- Current lactation status
- History of breastfeeding

✓   Medications and history of hormone therapy

✓   Family history, especially history of breast disease or ovarian cancer, age at onset, and relationship to the patient

✓   Carcinogen exposure, especially tobacco use, radiation exposure, and chemical exposure

Key Physical Findings

The breasts should be inspected visually with the patient in an upright position. The physician should note any asymmetry; obvious masses; nipple discharge; and skin changes, including rashes, dimpling, and inflammation. The physician should also note unilateral nipple retraction or inversion.

Each breast should be palpated, with the patient supine and one arm at a time raised above the patient's head.

Other physical features as follows should be evaluated:

✓   Characteristics of a benign breast lump

- Smooth
- Mobile
- Soft to firm
- Well-demarcated
- Symmetric thickening

- Changes with menstrual cycle
- No skin changes

✓ Characteristics of a worrisome breast mass

- Single lesion
- Firm or hard
- Immobile
- Size exceeding 2 cm
- Lack of tenderness to touch
- Ill-defined margins
- Skin or nipple retraction
- Erythema
- Edema of breast or affected arm
- Axillary or supraclavicular lymphadenopathy
- Fixation to chest wall or to surrounding skin
- Ulceration
- Asymmetric spontaneous bloody nipple discharge

Suggested Work-Up

See the algorithm in Figure 6-1 for the management of a palpable breast mass. The triple test is discussed in the introduction to this chapter.

In a young woman who presents with a breast lump and with a history and physical examination results that are not suggestive of malignancy, it is reasonable to recheck the lump about a week after the onset of menstruation. If it does not regress, she needs further work-up.

Clinical breast examination	Best performed by a clinician 1 week after menses
Imaging	
Mammography	Recommended for routine screening of all asymptomatic women 40 years and older
	Used for all women over age 40 with a solid mass, residual mass after cyst aspiration, or bloody fluid on cyst aspiration
Ultrasonography	Useful to differentiate between solid and cystic breast masses when a palpable breast mass is not well seen on a mammogram

Especially helpful in young women with dense breast tissue when a palpable mass is not visualized on a mammogram

Biopsy

FNA

A 20- to 25-gauge needle is used to aspirate cystic fluid or sample solid lesions for cytologic study; if there is bloody fluid, or no fluid, the fluid or cells should be sent for cytologic analysis

Often the first step in evaluating patients with palpable breast masses

Core-needle biopsy

A 14- to 18-gauge needle is used to sample a breast mass that is small or difficult to palpate

Produces a larger tissue sample than does FNA and may be used in conjunction with ultrasonography or stereotactic imaging for lesions that are small or difficult to palpate

May be used when FNA result is nondiagnostic, when FNA result is benign but mammography yields positive results, or when FNA result is atypical or suspect; also may be used when FNA reveals cystic fluid that is bloody or if there is residual mass after cyst aspiration

Useful in distinguishing atypical hyperplasia and ductal carcinoma in situ from invasive disease

Excisional biopsy

The "gold standard" for evaluating breast masses

Indicated in patients with clinically suspicious lesions and lesions in which results of imaging or tissue studies are equivocal

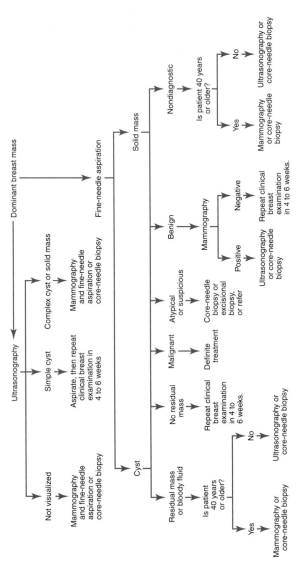

Figure 6-1. Diagnostic algorithm for patients with palpable breast masses. (*From Klein S: Evaluation of palpable breast masses. Am Fam Physician 2005;71:1731-1738.*)

Additional Work-Up

For women at very high risk for breast cancer, genetic testing may be offered. Women with *BRCA1* or *BRCA2* mutations have a lifetime risk of developing breast cancer as high as 85%. Patients with these gene mutations also have an elevated risk for ovarian, colon, prostate, and pancreatic cancers. Of all women with breast cancer, approximately 5% to 10% may have *BRCA1* or *BRCA2* mutations. Genetic testing may be considered for members of high-risk families. Genetic counseling before and after testing is recommended.

FURTHER READING

Apantaku LM: Breast cancer diagnosis and screening. Am Fam Physician 2000;62:596-602.

Esserman LJ: New approaches to the imaging, diagnosis, and biopsy of breast lesions. Cancer J 2002;8(Supp 1):S1-S14.

Klein S: Evaluation of palpable breast masses. Am Fam Physician 2005;71:1731-1738.

Morris KT, Pommier RF, Morris A, et al: Usefulness of the triple test score for palpable breast masses. Arch Surg 2001;136:1008-1012.

Morris KT, Vetto JT, Petty JK, et al: A new score for the evaluation of palpable breast masses in women under age 40. Am J Surg 2002;184:346-347.

Poggi MM, Harney KF: The breast. In DeCherney AH, Nathan L, Goodwin TM, eds: Current Obstetrics & Gynecologic Diagnosis & Treatment, 10th ed. New York: McGraw-Hill, 2007:621-630.

Pruthi S: Detection and evaluation of a palpable breast mass. Mayo Clin Proc 2001;76:641-648.

Steinberg JL, Trudeau ME, Ryder DE, et al: Combined fine-needle aspiration, physical examination and mammography in the diagnosis of palpable breast masses: their relation to outcome for women with primary breast cancer. Can J Surg 1996;39:302-311. [Erratum in Can J Surg 1997;40:9.]

Kathleen Dor

Breast pain, or mastalgia, is a very common complaint in women and represents the most common symptom in women seeking breast evaluation. Breast pain can be divided into three general categories: cyclic breast pain, noncyclic breast pain, and extramammary pain.

In young women, breast pain is usually cyclic, occurring most often a few days before menses and resolving after menses. Minor breast discomfort and swelling within the few days before the onset of menses is considered a normal physiologic occurrence. More severe and prolonged pain is considered cyclic mastalgia. Cyclic breast pain is usually bilateral and diffuse.

Noncyclic breast pain, in contrast, involves constant or intermittent pain that is not associated with the menstrual cycle. Noncyclic mastalgia is less common than cyclic mastalgia, is often unilateral, and often occurs postmenopausally. Noncyclic mastalgia often is described as "burning," "achy," or "sore."

Extramammary pain caused by various conditions may manifest as breast pain, although costochondritis represents the most common cause of extramammary pain. It is usually easy to distinguish between pain localized to the breast or chest wall and that radiating from elsewhere.

Many women who seek treatment for breast pain are concerned about breast cancer, although in the presence of normal examination findings and normal mammograms, the risk of breast cancer is very low. If the pain is mild, an appropriate evaluation is usually sufficient. However, in more severe cases, the mastalgia may interfere with usual daily activities, and treatment may be necessary to help alleviate the symptoms.

Medications That Can Cause Breast Pain

Antihypertensive and Cardiac Medications

Digoxin

Methyldopa

Minoxidil

Spironolactone

Reserpine

Antimicrobial Agents

Ketoconazole

Metronidazole

Hormonal Medications

Estrogens

Oral contraceptives

Progestogens

Psychiatric Medications

Amitriptyline

Chlordiazepoxide

Doxepin

Haloperidol

Selective serotonin reuptake inhibitors

Venlafaxine

Miscellaneous Agents

Carboprost

Cimetidine

Cyclosporine

Dinoprostone

Domperidone

Estramustine

Methadone

Penicillamine

Causes of Breast Pain

Cyclic Breast Pain

Noncyclic Breast Pain

Abscess or cellulitis

Benign tumors (such as fibroadenoma)

Breast cancer

Cysts

Mastitis

Medications

Pregnancy

Surgical procedures (postsurgical breast pain)

Trauma

Extramammary Pain

Biliary duct disease

Coronary artery disease

Esophageal spasm

Gastroesophageal reflux disease

Musculoskeletal pain

Neoplasm (such as lung cancer)

Neuropathic pain

Pericarditis

Pneumonia

Pulmonary embolus

Thoracic aortic aneurysm dissection

Key Historical Features

✓   Location, quality, timing (cyclic vs. noncyclic), relationship to exercise, and severity of the pain

✓   Associated symptoms such as redness, swelling, lump, or nipple discharge (can help focus the examination)

✓   Fever

✓   Weight loss

✓   Trauma

✓   Medications

✓   Medical history

  • A personal history of breast cancer, which increases a patient's risk for recurrent disease

  • Cardiac risk factors such as hypertension, hyperlipidemia, diabetes, and tobacco use

✓   Gynecologic and reproductive history

  • Early age at menarche, nulliparity, and pregnancy after age 30, which are associated with increased risk of breast cancer

  • Breastfeeding or recent childbirth, which increase risk for mastitis

  • Pregnancy, which may lead to breast pain

✓   Family history, especially of breast cancer and coronary artery disease

✓   Symptoms

  Cardiovascular

  • Chest pain caused by cardiac ischemia is often precipitated by exertion and relieved by rest. Patients often describe the pain as squeezing, tightening pressure. Patients may also experience dyspnea.

- Aortic dissection can cause a painful ripping sensation that radiates to the back and abdomen.

Pulmonary

- Shortness of breath can indicate coronary artery disease, pneumonia, or pulmonary embolism.
- Cough, either productive or nonproductive, may indicate pneumonia. A chronic cough can be associated with gastroesophageal reflux disease.

Gastrointestinal

- Chest pain caused by gastroesophageal reflux disease is often associated with meals and worsened with lying flat.
- Patients with biliary colic often complain of epigastric or right upper quadrant pain that radiates to the right shoulder. Patients may also experience chest pain. The pain often starts after a fatty meal, increases over an hour, and then lessens. The pain can be associated with vomiting.

Key Physical Findings

The physical examination should be guided by the history and may include the following evaluations:

✓ Assessment of vital signs

✓ General evaluation of health status

✓ Breast examination

- Both breasts should be visually inspected, with the patient upright and lying down. The physician should inspect for asymmetry, dimpling, retraction, or erythema of the skin and changes to the nipples.
- Both breasts should be palpated for masses, and both the axilla should be palpated for lymphadenopathy.

✓ Cardiopulmonary examination

- A thorough examination of the lungs and heart can help determine the cause of chest or breast pain.
- In order to perform an adequate examination of the chest wall, the patient should roll to the side so that the breast tissue moves out of the way.

✓ Abdominal examination for tenderness, distension, guarding, mass, organomegaly, or rebound

✓ Pelvic examination to evaluate for an ovarian tumor

Initial Work-Up

Mammography	If the pain is localized to the breast and if the patient is aged 30 years or older
Breast ultrasonography	Useful for evaluating for a mass at any age in patients with localized breast pain
Fine-needle aspiration or biopsy	Should be performed if a mass is palpated
Pregnancy test	If the patient is of childbearing age

Additional Work-Up

Radiography	If the pain is not localized to the breasts, chest radiography should be considered to evaluate the bony structures of the chest as well as the lungs and heart
	If the patient has had trauma and the pain is localized to other structures, obtain the appropriate x-ray, such as clavicle, rib, or shoulder
Electrocardiography	If the patient's pain is typical for cardiac pain or the patient has risk factors for coronary artery disease
Cardiac stress test	If the patient has typical chest pain or risk for cardiac disease; options include treadmill stress test, stress echocardiography, or cardiac nuclear perfusion scan
Abdominal ultrasonography	If the examination findings are suspect for cholecystitis

FURTHER READING

Millet AV, Dirbas FM: Clinical management of breast pain: a review. Obstet Gynecol Survey 2002;579:451-461.

Morrow M: The evaluation of common breast problems. Am Fam Physician 2000;61:2371-2378-2385.

Smith RL, Pruthi S, Fitzpatrick LA. Evaluation and management of breast pain. Mayo Clin Proc 2004;79:353-372.

Kathleen Dor

Breastfeeding has numerous benefits to the child and mother. Breastfed infants have lower rates of respiratory tract infections, otitis media, allergies, necrotizing enterocolitis, and serious bacterial infections. They also have lower rates of sudden infant death syndrome, diabetes, lymphoma, leukemia, obesity, hyperlipidemia, and asthma. Children who were breastfed also perform better on cognitive development tests. Benefits to the mother include decreased postpartum bleeding, increased temporal spacing between pregnancies, weight loss, lower risk of breast and ovarian cancer, and decreased risk of osteoporosis. In addition, breastfeeding results in less employee absenteeism, lower health care costs, and lower costs to families.

The American Academy of Pediatrics (AAP) and the American Academy of Family Physicians (AAFP) recommend that infants should be exclusively breastfed for the first 6 months and that breastfeeding continue through the first year of life. Promotion of breastfeeding can be achieved by encouragement and education before and after delivery, rooming in (in which mother and newborn share a hospital room), skin-to-skin contact after delivery, avoidance of supplements, avoidance of pacifiers until after breastfeeding is well-established, and follow-up with a health care provider when the infant is 3 to 5 days of age and 2 to 3 weeks of age.

Breastfeeding problems can sometimes result in serious consequences such as dehydration, failure to thrive, and jaundice in the infant. It is important that newborns and mothers have close follow-up after discharge from the hospital to prevent and identify these problems.

In a few cases, breastfeeding is contraindicated. Mothers with active untreated tuberculosis, positive human T cell lymphotrophic virus, or herpes lesions on their nipples should not breastfeed. Mothers who are being treated with radioactive isotopes or chemotherapy also should not breastfeed. In addition, infants with classic galactosemia should not be breastfed. In the United States, human immunodeficiency virus (HIV) infection is a contraindication to breastfeeding. Phenylalanine intake must be reduced if the mother or infant has PKU. Partial breastfeeding is often recommended.

Medications That May Inhibit Lactation

Ergotamine

Levodopa

Oral contraceptives

Thiazide diuretics

Causes of Breastfeeding Problems

Environmental Issues

Domestic violence

Early hospital discharge

Employment barriers

Hospital policies and practices that hinder breastfeeding

Poor postdischarge follow-up

Poor social support

Neonatal Causes

Cleft lip or cleft palate

Diseases such as cardiac disease or sepsis in the infant

Multiple infants

Poor latch-on or ineffective suck

Premature birth

Shortened frenulum

Maternal Causes

Alcohol consumption in moderate or large amounts

Blocked milk duct

Breast abscess

Breast engorgement

Breast surgeries, especially breast reduction

Candidal infection of the nipples

Delayed breastfeeding

Flat or inverted nipples

History of breast irradiation for cancer

Hypoplastic breasts

Illicit drug use

Inadequate frequency or length of each feeding

Interruption of breastfeeding

Lack of prenatal and postpartum education

Mastitis

Maternal disabilities, such as rheumatoid arthritis, cerebral palsy, and carpal tunnel syndrome

Maternal illness, such as hypothyroidism, gestational ovarian theca lutein cysts, or Sheehan syndrome

Maternal psychologic disease

Medications

Nipple pain or cracked nipples

Postoperative pain (after cesarean section)

Postpartum hemorrhage

Postpartum depression

Retained placenta

Smoking

Key Historical Features

✓   Birth history

- Apgar scores
- Infant birth weight
- Gestational age at birth
- Complications at delivery, such as shoulder dystocia or surgical delivery
- Neonatal complications, especially if infant required treatment in the neonatal intensive care unit or if invasive procedures, such as aggressive suctioning, were performed

✓   Maternal factors

- Pregnancy complications
- Medication use
- Alcohol use
- Smoking
- Illicit drug use
- History of eating disorders
- Inadequate diet/fluid intake
- History or symptoms of depression
- Experiences with breastfeeding during previous pregnancies
- Inadequate support system
- History of breast surgeries
- Type of breast pump, frequency of pumping, and amount of milk pumped per 24 hours
- Pain while breastfeeding
- Breast engorgement
- Use of nipple shields, which can decrease milk production
- Use of pacifiers, bottles, or formula

✓   Neonatal factors

- Amount of urination (three to five times per 24 hours by age 3 to 5 days and four to six times per 24 hours by age 5 to 7 days)
- Bowel movements (three or four stools per 24 hours by age 3 to 5 days and three to six stools per 24 hours by age 5 to 7 days)
- Weight gain (infant should return to birth weight by 2 weeks of age)
- Sleep schedule
- Frequency of breastfeeding and duration at each breast
- Amount of pumped breast milk consumed
- Alertness of infant during feeding

Key Physical Findings

During the examination, both the mother and infant should be examined. In addition, it is very useful to observe the mother breastfeeding her infant.

✓   Neonatal examination

- Naked weight before and after feeding to document amount of breast milk consumed and to compare with birth weight
- Signs of dehydration (dry mucous membranes, loss of skin turgor, depressed anterior fontanelle)
- Jaundice
- Sleepiness of infant during feeding
- Examination of the infant for cleft palate or tight frenulum
- Cardiovascular examination to evaluate for congenital cardiac disease

✓   Maternal examination

- Breasts should be evaluated for inverted/flat nipples, cracked/bleeding nipples, engorgement, mastitis, evidence of prior surgeries, and asymmetry
- Evaluation of the mother's mood for evidence of depression

✓   Breastfeeding technique

- Adequate latch-on (infant's mouth is wide open and covering the entire nipple and most of the areola)
- Position of the infant while breastfeeding (infant should be well supported with the chest and abdomen facing the mother's chest and the infant's mouth at the level of the nipple)
- Breast should be supported by mother with the "C-hold" (four fingers on underside of breast and thumb on top of breast)
- Swallowing sounds should be heard during feeding

Suggested Work-Up

In most cases, a careful documentation of history and physical examination, as well as observation of the mother breastfeeding, are adequate for managing breastfeeding difficulties. However, if the infant appears ill or significantly jaundiced, further work-up is necessary. Further work-up is also warranted if a low milk supply is thought to be caused by maternal illness.

Maternal Work-Up

Complete blood cell count	To detect anemia if milk supply appears low
Thyroid-stimulating hormone measurement	To detect hypothyroidism if milk supply appears low

Neonatal Work-Up

Total and direct bilirubin measurement	If significant jaundice is present
Complete blood cell count	If significant jaundice is present or if sepsis or infection is suspected
Blood cultures	If sepsis is suspected
Lumbar puncture	If sepsis is suspected
Urinalysis and urine culture	If sepsis is suspected

Additional Work-Up

Pelvic ultrasonography in mother	If retained placenta is suspected
Testosterone measurement	If gestational ovarian theca lutein cyst is suspected (testosterone level is elevated)

FURTHER READING

American Academy of Pediatrics: Breastfeeding and the use of human milk. Pediatrics 2005;115:496-506.

Amir LH: Breastfeeding: managing "supply" difficulties. Austral Fam Physician 2006;35: 686-689.

Breastfeeding and Maternal Medication: Recommendations for Drugs in the Eleventh WHO Model List of Essential Drugs. Geneva: World Health Organization, 2002.

Neifert MR: Breastmilk transfer: positioning, latch-on, and screening for problems in milk transfer. Clin Obstet Gynecol 2004;47:656-675.

Sinusas K: Initial management of breastfeeding. Am Fam Physician 2001;64:981-988.

Kathleen Dor

Chest pain is a very common complaint of patients presenting to the emergency room, as well as those presenting to outpatient clinics. More than 50% of patients presenting to the emergency department with chest pain have acute coronary syndrome, pulmonary embolism, or heart failure. However, most patients presenting to outpatient departments have diseases such as stable angina, musculoskeletal disorders, gastrointestinal disease, pulmonary disease, or psychiatric disorders.

Of patients who present with acute coronary syndrome, women are more likely than men to experience atypical chest pain and complain of associated symptoms such as nausea, vomiting, fatigue, dyspnea, or neck and shoulder pain. In addition, the diagnosis of acute coronary syndrome is more likely to be delayed in women. It is important that when a woman presents with chest pain, the history is carefully documented and a careful physical examination is performed to evaluate for more serious causes of chest pain. A complete work-up should be performed if it is indicated.

Medications Linked to Chest Pain

Azathioprine (pancreatitis)

Corticosteroids (pancreatitis)

Cyclosporine (pancreatitis)

Furosemide (pancreatitis)

Nonsteroidal anti-inflammatory drugs (NSAIDs) (peptic ulcer disease)

Oral contraceptives (pancreatitis, pulmonary embolism)

Sulfonamides (pancreatitis)

Tacrolimus (pancreatitis)

Tetracycline (pancreatitis)

Thiazides (pancreatitis)

Valproic acid (pancreatitis)

Causes of Chest Pain in Women

Breast Pain

Abscess

Breast cancer

Breast cyst

Cyclic breast pain

Mastitis

Cardiac Causes

Acute coronary syndrome (myocardial infarction, unstable angina)

Aortic stenosis

Coronary artery dissection

Coronary artery spasm

Heart failure

Myocarditis

Pericarditis

Stable angina

Thoracic aortic dissection (TAD)

Gastrointestinal Causes

Biliary disease

Esophageal cancer

Esophageal spasm

Gastric cancer

Gastroesophageal reflux disease

Pancreatic cancer

Pancreatitis

Peptic ulcer disease

Musculoskeletal Causes

Contusion

Costochondritis

Disk disease (cervical or thoracic)

Fibromyalgia

Osteoarthritis

Rib fracture

Thoracic outlet syndrome

Tietze syndrome

Psychiatric Causes

Depression

Factitious disorder

Panic disorder

Somatization

Pulmonary Causes

Bronchitis

Lung cancer

Pleuritis

Pneumonia

Pneumothorax

Pulmonary embolism

Other Causes

Familial Mediterranean fever

Herpes zoster

Mediastinal tumors

Key Historical Features

✓ Type of pain (pleuritic pain vs. nonpleuritic pain; crushing pain vs. sharp versus burning)

✓ Severity of pain

✓ Duration and onset of pain

✓ Location of pain

✓ Prior episodes of chest pain

✓ Exacerbating factors, especially exercise

✓ Relieving factors, especially rest or nitroglycerin

✓ Worsening of pain with certain movements

✓ Radiation of pain

✓ Relation of pain to meals

✓ History of trauma

✓ Fever

✓ Associated symptoms, especially cardiac symptoms

- Syncope
- Dizziness
- Weakness
- Palpitations

✓ Medical history

- Risk factors for coronary artery disease: diabetes, hyperlipidemia, hypertension, family history of coronary artery disease, smoking history

- History of coronary artery disease
- Review risk factors for pulmonary embolism: use of oral contraceptives, hormone replacement therapy, hypercoagulable state (malignancies, thrombophilia, pregnancy, recent surgery, recent travel, immobilization
- Review risk factors for thoracic aortic dissection: hypertension, Marfan syndrome, cocaine use

✓ Obstetric/gynecologic history

- Evaluate possibility of pregnancy, which affects the work-up results and treatment

✓ Surgical history

✓ Medications

✓ History of recreational drug use, smoking, alcohol use

✓ Family history

✓ Review of systems

- Cardiac (see earlier description)
- Gastrointestinal
  — Nausea and vomiting
  — Rectal bleeding
  — Abdominal pain
- Pulmonary
  — Cough (may be a sign of pneumonia, lung cancer, heart failure, or bronchitis)
  — Hemoptysis (may be a sign of pneumonia, lung cancer, pulmonary embolism, or heart failure)
  — Dyspnea (may be a sign of acute coronary syndrome, heart failure, pneumonia, pulmonary embolism, or pneumothorax)
- Neurologic
  — Patient should be evaluated for weakness or numbness resulting from a stroke, which can be caused by TAD
- Psychiatric
  — History of depression or anxiety should be sought; however, symptoms should not be presumed to be a manifestation of psychiatric illness

Key Physical Findings

✓ Evaluation of vital signs, including pulse oximetry

✓ General assessment of well-being

✓ Cardiovascular examination for rhythm, rate, murmurs, heart sounds, apical impulse, peripheral pulses, and jugular venous distension

✓ Pulmonary examination for the presence of abnormal lung sounds, egophony, or dullness to percussion

✓ Abdominal examination for tenderness, organomegaly, or masses

✓ Rectal examination to evaluate for bleeding

✓ Neurologic examination for evidence of a stroke

✓ Skin examination for evidence of herpes zoster

✓ Musculoskeletal examination for evidence of chest wall, neck, or shoulder tenderness

✓ Extremity examination for evidence of deep vein thrombosis

Suggested Work-Up

In some patients, an adequate documentation of history and a physical examination may be enough to determine that a patient has a nonthreatening cause of chest pain. However, most patients require at least electrocardiography, chest radiography, and selected laboratory tests.

Electrocardiography	To evaluate for evidence of ischemia, pericarditis, pulmonary embolism, arrhythmias, or heart failure
Chest radiography	To evaluate for pulmonary disease, heart failure, or TAD
Serum markers of myocardial damage (creatine kinase, isoenzyme of creatine kinase with muscle and brain subunits (CK-MB), troponin T, troponin I)	To evaluate for acute coronary syndrome

Additional Work-Up

Complete blood cell count	To evaluate for infection or anemia
Amylase and/or lipase measurement	If pancreatitis is suspected
Aspartate transaminase (AST), alanine transaminase (ALT), and bilirubin measurement	If liver or biliary disease is suspected

Abdominal ultrasonography	If liver or biliary disease is suspected
Upper endoscopy	If peptic ulcer or gastric cancer is suspected
Mammography	If a breast mass is palpated or the patient is due for breast cancer screening
Commuted tomographic (CT) scan of chest	If pulmonary embolism, TAD, or lung cancer is suspected
D-Dimer	When used in conjunction with scoring systems, a normal D-dimer, along with a low pretest probability of a deep vein thrombosis or pulmonary embolism, can be used to safely withhold further evaluation such as lower extremity compression ultrasonography, ventilation-perfusion scanning, or CT angiography
Ventilation perfusion scanning or CT angiography	If pulmonary embolism is suspected
Cardiac stress testing	If coronary artery disease is suspected
CT scanning of abdomen	If an intra-abdominal malignancy, abscess, or other disease process is suspected
Arterial blood gas measurements	If the patient is hypoxic or has evidence of significant pulmonary disease
Blood cultures	If an infectious process is suspected
Sputum cultures	If pneumonia is suspected
Echocardiography	If heart failure, pericarditis, valvular disease, or other cardiac disease processes are suspected
Rib series (radiography)	May be considered if rib fracture is suspected
Brain natriuretic peptide measurement	If heart failure is suspected

| Venous compression ultrasonography | To evaluate for deep vein thrombosis in a patient who may have a pulmonary embolism |

FURTHER READING

Boie ET: Initial evaluation of chest pain. Emerg Med Clin North Am 2005;23:937-957.

Butler KH, Swencki SA: Chest pain: a clinical assessment. Radiol Clin North Am 2006;44:165-179.

Cayley WE: Diagnosing the cause of chest pain. Am Fam Physician 2005;72:2012-2021.

Douglas PS, Ginsburg GS: The evaluation of chest pain in women. N Engl J Med 1996;334:1311-1315.

Goldman L, Ausiello D, eds: Cecil Textbook of Medicine, 2nd ed. Philadelphia: Elsevier, 2004.

Pilote L, Dasgupta K, Guru V, et al: A comprehensive view of sex-specific issues related to cardiovascular disease. CMAJ 2007;176(6 Suppl):S1-S44. [Erratum in CMAJ 2007;176(9):1310.]

Kathleen Dor

In girls, puberty begins with the development of breast buds, which is controlled by estrogens that are produced by the ovaries. This is followed by the appearance of pubic and axillary hair, which is controlled by androgens that are produced by the adrenal cortex and the ovaries. In addition, there is rapid skeletal growth. Menarche is a late occurrence in puberty.

A patient should be evaluated for delayed puberty if she has not had any breast development by age 13 years or if there is more than a 5-year delay between the initial development of breasts and menarche. Delayed puberty should be classified as constitutional delay, hypogonadotropic hypogonadism (low gonadotropin levels resulting from hypothalamic-pituitary failure), or hypergonadotropic hypogonadism (resulting from gonadal failure with high gonadotropin levels).

Medications Linked to Delayed Puberty

Chemotherapeutic agents

Chronic corticosteroids

Causes of Delayed Puberty

Constitutional Delayed Puberty

Hypogonadotropic Hypogonadism

Brain trauma

Chemotherapy

Congenital hypopituitarism

Central nervous system (CNS) tumors and infiltrative diseases

- Astrocytoma
- Craniopharyngioma
- Glioma
- Histiocytosis X
- Prolactinoma

Excessive exercise

Genetic defects

- Kallmann syndrome
- Leptin receptor deficiency

Marijuana use

Post—CNS infection disease

Radiation therapy

Syndromes

- CHARGE syndrome (coloboma, heart disease, atresia choanae, retarded growth and retarded development and/or anomalies, genital hypoplasia, and ear anomalies and/or deafness)
- Gaucher disease
- Lawrence-Moon-Bardet-Biedl syndrome
- LEOPARD syndrome (lentigines, electrocardiographic abnormalities, ocular hypertelorism, pulmonary stenosis, abnormal genitalia, retardation of growth, deafness)
- Prader-Willi syndrome

Systemic illness

- Acquired immunodeficiency syndrome (AIDS)
- Anorexia nervosa or bulimia
- Asthma
- Celiac disease
- Chronic kidney disease
- Cushing syndrome
- Cystic fibrosis
- Diabetes mellitus
- Growth hormone deficiency
- Hemosiderosis
- Hyperprolactinemia
- Hypothyroidism
- Inflammatory bowel disease
- Juvenile rheumatoid arthritis
- Malnutrition
- Neoplasms
- Sickle-cell disease
- Thalassemia

Hypergonadotropic Hypogonadism

Androgen insensitivity

Autoimmune oophoritis

Biosynthetic defects

Chemotherapy

Galactosemia

Gonadal dysgenesis

Noonan syndrome

Radiation therapy

Turner syndrome

Key Historical Features

✓ Age at which breasts started developing and when pubic and axillary hair appeared

✓ Growth history

✓ Developmental history

✓ Dietary and exercise history

✓ Mood changes associated with puberty

✓ Anosmia (Kallmann syndrome)

✓ Deafness (gonadal dysgenesis)

✓ History or symptoms of chronic diseases (see items listed earlier), as well as use of corticosteroids

✓ Medical history, especially of chronic diseases, eating disorders, congenital heart disease, chemotherapy, or radiation therapy

✓ Surgical history

✓ Medications

✓ Family history of delayed puberty, genetic disorders, or neurologic disorders

Key Physical Findings

✓ Height and weight plotted on a growth curve

✓ Evaluation for any dysmorphic features

✓ Manifestations of Turner syndrome (short stature, webbed neck, broad chest with widely spaced nipples, ptosis)

✓ Manifestations of Noonan syndrome (short stature, triangular face, low-set ears, pectus excavatum, short webbed neck)

✓ Ophthalmologic examination for visual field defects, which may indicate a pituitary tumor

✓ Cardiovascular examination for any congenital heart defects (Noonan syndrome, LEOPARD syndrome, Turner syndrome, or CHARGE syndrome)

✓ Determination of stage of breast development

✓ Gynecologic examination of genitalia for pubertal stage and appropriateness to gender

✓ Dermatologic examination for pubic and axillary hair, as well as acne

✓ Neurologic examination

Suggested Work-Up

Radiography of left wrist	To assess bone age
Luteinizing hormone (LH) and follicle-stimulating hormone (FSH) measurements	To distinguish a hypothalamic-pituitary cause or constitutional delay (low levels) from a gonadal cause (high levels)
Cortisol level measurement	To evaluate pituitary function
Insulin-like growth factor I measurement	To evaluate pituitary function
Estradiol	To evaluate for gonadal failure
Complete blood cell count	To evaluate for anemia of chronic disease
Liver function tests	To evaluate for chronic liver disease
Creatinine measurement	To evaluate for chronic renal disease
Electrolyte measurements	To evaluate for metabolic disorders and chronic renal disease
Thyroid-stimulating hormone (TSH) and free thyroxine (T4) measurement	To evaluate for thyroid disease
Fasting blood glucose measurement	To evaluate for diabetes
Urinalysis	To evaluate for renal disease

Additional Work-Up

Erythrocyte sedimentation rate measurement	To evaluate for inflammatory processes

Celiac disease panel: tissue transglutaminase antibody, gliadin antibody, and endomysial antibody	If celiac disease is suspected
Prolactin measurement	To evaluate for hyperprolactinemia
Karyotype analysis	If a chromosomal abnormality is suspected
Sigmoidoscopy	If inflammatory bowel disease is suspected
Magnetic resonance imaging (MRI) of brain and pituitary gland	If a disorder of the hypothalamic-pituitary axis is suspected
Pelvic ultrasonography	If an abnormality of the uterus or ovaries is suspected
Gonadotropin-releasing hormone (GnRH) stimulation test	To evaluate the hypothalamic-pituitary-gonadal axis

FURTHER READING

Argente J: Diagnosis of late puberty. Horm Res 1999;51(Supp. 3):95-100.

Blondell RD, Foster MB, Dave KC: Disorders of puberty. Am Fam Physician 1999;60(1):209-218223-224.

Chapman AJ: Delayed puberty. BMJ 1985;290:1493-1496.

Grumbach MM, Styne DM: Puberty: ontogeny, neuroendocrinology, physiology and disorders. In Larsen PR, Kronenberg HM, Melmed S, et al, eds: Williams Textbook of Endocrinology, 11th ed, Philadelphia: Saunders, 2008, pp 969-1104.

Nathan BM, Palmert MR: Regulation and disorder of pubertal timing. Endocrinol Metab Clin North Am 2005;34:617-641.

11 DYSPAREUNIA

Kathleen Dor

Dyspareunia is recurrent genital pain during or after sexual intercourse. The pain may occur in the more superficial structures, such as the vulva, or deeper in the pelvic structures. Although dyspareunia occurs in both men and women, it is more prevalent in women. Dyspareunia may occur in as many as 60% of women, although far fewer seek medical care for this problem. Dyspareunia often has multiple causes, including both physical and psychologic causes.

Patients with dyspareunia may complain of a well-defined and localized pain, or they may express a general disinterest in and dissatisfaction with intercourse that results from the associated discomfort. The most common pain with dyspareunia occurs during coitus, but some women experience pain afterward, and others report pain at both times. Dyspareunia is differentiated from vaginismus and from problems resulting from inadequate lubrication.

The *Diagnostic and Statistical Manual of Mental Disorders*, 4th edition (DSM-IV), defines dyspareunia as a sexual pain disorder, a subcategory of sexual dysfunction. However, the biopsychosocial approach emphasizes that physical and psychologic factors may be instigating causes and reasons for perpetuation of the symptoms. The causes of women's sexual pain differ for each subtype of pain, with substantial overlap between types of pain. What remains the most unclear is the cause of the original sensitization.

Medications Linked to Dyspareunia

Bromocriptine mesylate (which can cause painful clitoral tumescence)

Cevimeline

Desipramine hydrochloride (which can cause painful orgasm)

Goserelin

Letrozole (which can cause vaginal dryness)

Leuprolide

Risperidone (which can cause vaginal dryness)

Causes of Dyspareunia

Anxiety

Arousal disorders

Bartholin gland abscess

Behçet syndrome

Bladder neoplasm

Breastfeeding

Cervical cancer

Chronic constipation

Contact dermatitis

Depression

Diverticular disease

Endometriosis

Endometritis

Hemorrhoids

Herpes infection

Hymenal stenosis

Hypertrophic vulvar dystrophy

Inadequate vaginal lubrication

Inflammatory bowel disease

Interstitial cystitis

Lichen sclerosis

Medications

Ovarian cysts

Ovarian neoplasms

Ovarian remnant syndrome

Pelvic congestion syndrome

Pelvic inflammatory disease

Postpartum dyspareunia

Postsurgical pain

Trauma

Urethral diverticulum

Urethritis

Urinary tract infection

Uterine fibroids

Uterine neoplasm

Vaginal agenesis

Vaginal duplication

Vaginal scarring

Vaginal septum

Vaginismus

Vaginitis

Vulvar neoplasms

Vulvar vestibulitis

Key Historical Features

✓ Gynecologic

- Location and timing of pain with relation to sexual intercourse
  — Pain with arousal may indicate Bartholin gland cyst swelling.
  — Pain of the external genitalia may indicate vulvitis or vestibulitis.
  — Pain with initial penile penetration may indicate vaginismus, vaginitis, vaginal/vulvar atrophy, vaginal/vulvar scarring, inadequate vaginal lubrication, or vaginal septation.
  — Midvaginal pain may indicate interstitial cystitis or urethritis.
  — Deep pain may indicate pelvic inflammatory disease, endometriosis, uterine fibroids, inflammatory bowel disease, or a pelvic mass.
- Quality and severity of pain
- Associated pruritus or vaginal discharge, which may indicate vaginitis or sexually transmitted diseases
- Timing of onset of pain (patients with pain since their first sexual experience may have a psychological cause, whereas patients with more recently acquired dyspareunia are more likely to have a physical cause)
- History of sexually transmitted diseases
- History of trauma, including that occurring during childbirth
- History of gynecologic surgery or irradiation
- Contraceptive method, especially intrauterine device
- Difficulty with lubrication or arousal

✓ Gastrointestinal

- Associated diarrhea, bleeding, or abdominal pain, which may indicate inflammatory bowel disease or diverticular disease
- Chronic constipation

✓ Genitourinary

- Dysuria, urinary urgency, or frequency, which may indicate interstitial cystitis or infection
- Hematuria, which may indicate bladder neoplasm or infection
- A history of recurrent urinary tract infections associated with negative culture results, which may indicate interstitial cystitis

✓ Skin
  • Use of new lotions or creams
  • History of skin diseases such as atopic dermatitis or psoriasis
✓ Psychologic
  • History of sexual or physical abuse
  • Symptoms of depression and anxiety

Key Physical Findings

✓ Gynecologic examination
  • Inspection of the external genitalia for tenderness, erythema, or any lesions
  • Examination of the external genitalia with a cotton swab for superficial tenderness; tenderness of the vulvar vestibule indicates vestibulitis
  • Vaginal examination with one finger to palpate the walls of the vagina, as well as the bladder and urethra, and evaluation of the tone of the pelvic floor muscles and voluntary muscle control
  • Speculum examination with a narrow speculum that is lubricated, to examine the vaginal mucosa and cervix
  • Bimanual examination to evaluate for cervical motion tenderness, adnexal or uterine tenderness, or any masses or nodules
✓ Gastrointestinal examination
  • Palpation of the abdomen for any tenderness, masses, or organomegaly
  • Rectal examination to evaluate for any masses

Suggested Work-Up

Pap smear	To evaluate for cervical dysplasia
Wet mount	To evaluate for vaginitis
Cervical culture/swab for gonorrhea and chlamydia	To evaluate for infection with *Neisseria gonorrhoeae* or *Chlamydia* organisms
Urinalysis and urine culture	To evaluate for urinary tract infection

Additional Work-Up

Herpesvirus culture	If lesions indicative of herpes are visualized

Pelvic ultrasonography	If a pelvic mass is palpated
Computed tomography of the pelvis or abdomen	If a pelvic or abdominal mass is palpated
Colposcopy	If a cervical lesion is visualized
Biopsy	If a vulvar, vaginal, or cervical lesion is visualized
Cystoscopy	If interstitial cystitis is suspected
Laparoscopy	If endometriosis is suspected
Flexible sigmoidoscopy or colonoscopy	If a colonic source of pain is suspected

FURTHER READING

American Psychiatric Association: Diagnostic and Statistical Manual of Mental Disorders, 4th ed. Washington, DC: American Psychiatric Association, 1994:511-518.

Canavan TP, Heckman CD: Dyspareunia in women: breaking the silence is the first step toward treatment. Postgrad Med 2000;108(2):149-166.

Carey JC: Pharmacological effects on sexual function. Obstet Gynecol Clin North Am 2006;33:599-620.

Heim LJ: Evaluation and differential diagnosis of dyspareunia. Am Fam Physician 2001;63:1535–1544, 1551-1552.

MacNeill C: Dyspareunia. Obstet Gynecol Clin North Am 2006;33:565-577.

Theodore O'Connell

Dysuria is the sensation of burning, pain, or discomfort on urination, most often the result of infection or inflammation of the bladder, the urethra, or both. Infection may manifest as urethritis, cystitis, or pyelonephritis. Although dysuria often is equated with urinary tract infection, dysuria also may result from vaginitis, malformations of the urinary tract, malignancy, hormonal conditions, trauma, interstitial cystitis, neurogenic conditions, and psychogenic disorders.

The timing of the dysuria may help pinpoint the location of the problem in the urinary tract. Discomfort at the start of urination suggests a urethral source of inflammation, whereas pain occurring over the suprapubic area upon completion of urination often indicates inflammation of the bladder.

Medications and Supplements Linked to Dysuria

Cantharidin
Cyclophosphamide
Dopamine
Penicillin G
Pumpkin seeds
Saw palmetto
Ticarcillin

Causes of Dysuria

Anatomic issues
- Bladder diverticula
- Urethral stricture

Infection
- Cervicitis
- Cystitis
- Urethritis
- Vulvovaginitis

Hormonal causes
- Vaginal/vulvar tissue atrophy and dryness in postmenopausal women

71

Inflammatory disorders
- Autoimmune disorders
- Behçet syndrome
- Reiter syndrome

Medication and supplement side effects

Neoplasm
- Bladder cancer
- Renal cell tumor
- Vaginal cancer
- Vulvar malignancy

Psychogenic disorders
- Anxiety
- Chemical dependency
- Chronic pain syndromes
- Depression
- Somatization
- Stress

Trauma
- Urethral instrumentation or catheter placement
- Urethral trauma during intercourse

Other causes
- Bicycle riding
- Horseback riding
- Interstitial cystitis
- Sensitivity to creams, sprays, soaps, or toilet paper
- Stones (renal, ureteral, and bladder)
- Urethral syndrome

Key Historical Features

✓ Onset and duration of dysuria

✓ Fever, chills, nausea, or vomiting

✓ Timing of dysuria, particularly if related to menstrual cycle

✓ Frequency of dysuria

✓ Severity

✓ Location of discomfort

✓ External versus internal dysuria

✓ Pain at onset of urination versus suprapubic pain after voiding

✓   Presence of hematuria

✓   Urinary frequency, urgency, or hesitation

✓   Nocturia

✓   Sexual habits

✓   Vaginal discharge

✓   Dyspareunia

✓   Use of topical irritants such as lubricants, douches, or soaps

✓   Back pain

✓   Joint pain

✓   Ocular symptoms

✓   Oral mucosal symptoms

✓   Medical history

✓   Surgical history

✓   Sexual history, including history of sexually transmitted diseases

✓   Tobacco use

✓   Medications

✓   Family history

Key Physical Findings

✓   Fever

✓   Head and neck examination for conjunctivitis or oral ulcers

✓   Abdominal examination to assess the kidneys and bladder

✓   Back examination for costovertebral angle tenderness

✓   Pelvic examination

✓   Digital rectal examination

✓   Inguinal lymphadenopathy

✓   Extremity examination for joint swelling or tenderness

✓   Skin examination for rash

Suggested Work-Up

Urinalysis	To evaluate for pyuria or hematuria
Urine culture	To accurately diagnose infection and determine antimicrobial susceptibility of infecting bacteria

Vaginal wet mount preparation	To detect infection with *Trichomonas vaginalis* and *Candida* species
Urethral smear or urine ligase chain reaction and polymerase chain reaction tests for *Neisseria gonorrhoeae* and *Chlamydia trachomatis*	To detect gonorrhea and chlamydia

Additional Work-Up

Urine cytologic testing	If urinary tract malignancy is suspected
Cystoscopy	To detect bladder or urethral pathology and confirm the diagnosis of interstitial cystitis; used in the evaluation of noninfectious hematuria
Renal ultrasonography	If kidney or ureter disease such as abscess or hydronephrosis is suspected
Bladder ultrasonography	If bladder or urethral stones are suspected or if bladder diverticula are suspected
Plain films of kidneys, ureters, and bladder	For rapid evaluation of suspected renal stones
Computed tomographic (CT) scan with contrast media (preferred)	To visualize avascular structure such as infarcts, cysts, abscesses, and necrotic tumors
CT scan without contrast media	To evaluate for renal stones/calcifications and to evaluate solid tissue in the urinary tract
Voiding cystourethrography	To assess for abnormalities such as vesicoureteral reflux, neurogenic bladder, urethral strictures, and diverticula
Intravenous pyelography	To evaluate recurrent urinary tract infection or localize ureteral calculi

| Magnetic resonance imaging (MRI) with gadolinium enhancement | To identify urinary obstruction or mass in patients with renal insufficiency or allergy to iodinated contrast media |

FURTHER READING

Bremnor JD, Sadovsky R: Evaluation of dysuria in adults. Am Fam Physician 2002;65:1589-1596.

Roberts RG, Hartlaub PP: Evaluation of dysuria in men. Am Fam Physician 1999;60:865-872.

Thomas A, Woodard C, Rovner ES, et al: Urologic complications of nonneurologic medications. Urol Clin North Am 2003;30:123-131.

13 FATIGUE

Theodore O'Connell

Fatigue is defined as a subjective state of sustained lack of energy or exhaustion with a decreased capacity for physical and mental work, which persists despite sufficient rest. Fatigue is one of the most common complaints in adults presenting for primary care in the United States and must be differentiated from weakness or exertional difficulties.

Acute viral syndromes are a common cause of fatigue and are usually self-limited. Fatigue that persists longer than 1 month generally warrants investigation. Although fatigue is usually the symptom of which the patient complains, careful history documentation often reveals associated symptoms. A targeted physical examination may lead to additional diagnostic clues. A laboratory examination may not be required in all cases of fatigue, but targeted testing may help the clinician pinpoint the cause of the patient's symptoms.

Depression is the most common cause of clinically important fatigue in patients presenting for primary care. Fatigue is common in the elderly population and may represent part of the normal aging process. However, fatigue should not be attributed to advanced age alone. Rather, fatigue as a consequence of advanced age should be a diagnosis of exclusion.

Medications Associated with Fatigue

Almost every medication may cause fatigue and should be considered in the evaluation of the patient with fatigue. The following categories of medications are more common causes of fatigue.

Antihistamines

Benzodiazepines

β Blockers

Blood pressure medications

Diuretics

Glucocorticoids

Narcotic pain medications

Nonsteroidal anti-inflammatory drugs (NSAIDs)

Selective serotonin reuptake inhibitors

Sleeping medications

Tricyclic antidepressants

Causes of Fatigue

Addison disease

Advancing age

Alcohol abuse

Allergic rhinitis

Amebiasis

Anemia

Anorexia nervosa

Bipolar disorder

Blastomycosis

Bulimia nervosa

Cancer

Carbon monoxide poisoning

Chemotherapy

Chronic pulmonary disease

Chronic sinusitis

Coccidioidomycosis

Cushing disease

Cytomegalovirus infection

Dementia

Depression

Dermatomyositis

Diabetes

Domestic abuse

Drug abuse

Endocarditis

Epstein-Barr virus infection

Fibromyalgia

Giardiasis

Heart failure

Heavy metal exposure

Helminth infestation

Hepatitis B or C

Histoplasmosis

Hypercalcemia

Hyperthyroidism

Hypothyroidism

Liver disease

Lyme disease

Lymphoma

Malnutrition

Medications

Mixed connective tissue disease

Multiple sclerosis

Myasthenia gravis

Obesity

Occult malignancy

Parkinson disease

Parvovirus B19 infection

Polymyalgia rheumatica

Polymyositis

Radiation therapy

Rheumatoid arthritis

Sarcoidosis

Significant weight loss

Situational stress

Sjögren syndrome

Sleep apnea

Systemic lupus erythematosus

Temporal arteritis

Toxin exposure

Tuberculosis

Uremia

Viral infections

Key Historical Features

✓ Onset

✓ Nature of the fatigue

✓ Medical history, including psychiatric history

✓ Medications

✓ Family history

✓ Social history

  • Travel

  • Alcohol use

- Drug use
- Dietary habits
- Caffeine consumption
- Life events or stressors, relationships with family members

✓ Systemic signs and symptoms

- Fever, chills
- Night sweats
- Weight loss or weight gain
- Appetite
- Arthralgias
- Myalgias
- Headache
- Adenopathy
- Paresthesias
- Sore throat
- Rash
- Sleep disturbance
- Anhedonia
- Weakness
- Problems with memory or concentration

Key Physical Findings

✓ Age

✓ Gender

✓ Weight

✓ Vital signs

✓ Head and neck examination for signs of anemia, sinusitis, oral ulcerations, postnasal drip, thyromegaly, or lymphadenopathy

✓ Ophthalmologic examination for signs of increased intracranial pressure, retinopathy, or anemia

✓ Cardiovascular examination, including jugular venous distension

✓ Pulmonary examination

✓ Abdominal examination for abdominal masses, hepatomegaly, splenomegaly, or ascites

✓ Examination of the musculature for signs of weakness or muscle atrophy

- ✓ Skin examination for color changes, rash, skin texture changes, or hair changes
- ✓ Pelvic examination
- ✓ Rectal examination, including that for stool guaiac
- ✓ Neurologic examination

Suggested Work-Up

Serial weight measurement	To help evaluate for depression or systemic illness
Monitoring of temperature	To help evaluate for infection or malignancy
Complete blood cell count (CBC)	To evaluate for infection or malignancy
Electrolyte measurements	To evaluate for adrenal insufficiency
Blood urea nitrogen (BUN) and creatinine measurements	To evaluate for renal failure
Glucose measurement	To evaluate for diabetes mellitus
Alanine transaminase (ALT) and aspartate transaminase (AST) measurements	To evaluate for hepatocellular disease
Total bilirubin measurement	To evaluate for hepatitis or hemolysis
Albumin measurement	To evaluate for malnutrition and hepatic synthetic dysfunction
Alkaline phosphatase measurement	To evaluate for obstructive liver disease
Creatine kinase measurement	To evaluate for muscle disease
Calcium measurement	To help detect hyperparathyroidism, cancer, and sarcoidosis
Phosphorus measurement	To evaluate for hypo- or hyperphosphatemia
Erythrocyte sedimentation rate (ESR) measurement	To help detect collagen-vascular disease, malignancy, endocarditis,

abscess, osteomyelitis, tuberculosis, and so forth

Thyroid-stimulating hormone (TSH) measurement

To evaluate for hyperthyroidism and hypothyroidism

Urinalysis

To evaluate for proteinuria and renal disease

Additional Work-Up

Lyme serologic profiles

If Lyme disease is suspected

Human immunodeficiency virus (HIV) testing

If the patient is at risk for HIV infection

Antinuclear antibody measurements (ANA)

If lupus or other collagen vascular diseases are suspected

Hepatitis B and C screening

If the patient is at risk of hepatitis B or C or if the patient has abnormal liver function test results

Purified protein derivative (PPD) skin test

If the patient is at risk for tuberculosis or if tuberculosis is suspected clinically

Chest radiography

If cardiopulmonary disease is suspected

Brucella titers

If brucellosis is suspected clinically

Monospot test or Epstein-Barr virus titers

If mononucleosis or Epstein-Barr infection is suspected

Cytomegalovirus (CMV) titers

If CMV infection is suspected

Blood cultures

If endocarditis or bacteremia is suspected

Histoplasma antigen measurement

If histoplasmosis is suspected

Adrenocorticotropic hormone (ACTH) test

If Cushing disease is suspected clinically

Tensilon test

If myasthenia gravis is suspected clinically

Echocardiography	If heart failure is suspected
Parvovirus immunoglobulin M (IgM) test	If parvovirus infection is suspected
Twenty-four-hour urine test for heavy metals	If heavy metal exposure is suspected
Serum angiotensin-converting enzyme (ACE) level	If sarcoidosis is suspected

FURTHER READING

Cho WK, Stollerman GH: Chronic fatigue syndrome. Hosp Pract (Off Ed) 1992;27(9): 221-224, 227-230.

Craig T, Kakumanu S: Chronic fatigue syndrome: evaluation and treatment. Am Fam Physician 2002;65:1083-1090.

Manzullo EF, Escalante CP: Research into fatigue. Hematol Oncol Clin North Am 2002: 619-628.

Morrison RE, Keating HJ: Fatigue in primary care. Obstet Gynecol Clin 2001;28:225-240.

GALACTORRHEA

Theodore O'Connell

Galactorrhea is the inappropriate production of milk from the breast in the absence of pregnancy or beyond 6 to 12 months post partum in a nonbreastfeeding woman. The discharge of milk may be unilateral or bilateral, may be intermittent or persistent, and may vary in volume. Galactorrhea may also occur in boys and men and in infants and teenage girls.

Distinguishing galactorrhea from other forms of nipple discharge is usually straightforward. In galactorrhea, the discharge has the appearance of milk, occurs from multiple ducts in the nipple, most commonly occurs bilaterally, and is usually spontaneous.

When nipple discharge is consistent with galactorrhea, the medical history often reveals the cause. Important elements of the history and physical examination are outlined in the following sections.

Medications Linked to Galactorrhea

Amphetamines
Butyrophenones
Calcium channel blockers
Cimetidine
Codeine
Methyldopa
Metoclopramide
Morphine
Oral contraceptives
Phenothiazines
Prochlorperazine
Reserpine
Risperidone
Selective serotonin reuptake inhibitors
Tricyclic antidepressants

Causes of Galactorrhea

Bronchogenic carcinoma
Chronic renal failure
Estrogen withdrawal

Heroin use

Hypothalamic lesions

- Craniopharyngioma
- Empty sella syndrome
- Pituitary stalk lesions
- Primary hypothalamic tumor
- Sarcoidosis
- Tuberculosis

Hypothyroidism

Idiopathic

Medications

Neonatal galactorrhea

Neurogenic causes

- Breast stimulation
- Burns
- Chest surgery
- Shingles

Pituitary tumors (usually prolactinoma)

Thoracic neoplasms

Key Historical Features

✓ Duration of galactorrhea

✓ Unilateral or bilateral presence

✓ Associated mass

✓ Medications

✓ Medical history, particularly thyroid disorders or renal failure

✓ Surgical history, especially recent chest surgery

✓ Family history, especially thyroid disorders or multiple endocrine neoplasia, which increase the risk for galactorrhea

✓ Reproductive history

- Oral contraceptives, the most common medication-related cause of galactorrhea
- Oligomenorrhea, amenorrhea, infertility, or decreased libido, suggestive of hyperprolactinemia
- Amenorrhea, which may indicate pregnancy or pituitary tumor

✓ Constitutional symptoms

- Fatigue and cold intolerance, suggestive of hypothyroidism
- Nervousness, heat intolerance, unusual sweating, and weight loss despite a normal or increased appetite, suggestive of thyrotoxicosis
- Polyuria and polydipsia, suggestive of pituitary or hypothalamic disease

✓ Skin symptoms

- Dry skin, suggestive of hypothyroidism
- Acne and hirsutism, suggestive of hyperandrogenism

✓ Gastrointestinal symptoms

- Constipation, suggestive of hypothyroidism

✓ Neurologic symptoms

- Headache, visual disturbance, and seizure, suggestive of pituitary or hypothalamic disease

Key Physical Findings

✓ Vital signs

✓ Poor growth or short stature, suggestive of hypothyroidism, hypopituitarism, or chronic renal failure

✓ Acromegaly or gigantism, suggestive of pituitary tumor

✓ Breast examination for nodules and discharge and determination of whether the discharge is from one or multiple ducts

✓ Cardiac examination for bradycardia suggestive of hypothyroidism or tachycardia suggestive of thyrotoxicosis

✓ Skin examination for dry skin, coarse hair, and myxedema, suggestive of hypothyroidism, or for hirsutism and acne, suggestive of hyperandrogenism

✓ Head and neck examination for goiter, suggestive of hypothyroidism

✓ Eye examination for visual field defect or papilledema, suggestive of pituitary tumor or intracranial mass

✓ Neurologic examination for hand tremor, suggestive of thyrotoxicosis, or for a cranial neuropathy, suggestive of pituitary tumor or intracranial mass

Suggested Work-Up

The evaluation of galactorrhea should proceed in a stepwise manner and be guided by findings from the history and physical examination.

Pregnancy test	To evaluate for pregnancy in women of childbearing age
Serum prolactin measurement	To evaluate for pituitary adenoma
Thyroid-stimulating hormone (TSH)	To evaluate for hypo- or hyperthyroidism

Additional Work-Up

If hyperprolactinemia is confirmed, medications that may cause elevation in prolactin levels should be withheld if possible. The prolactin level should then be measured again.

If true hyperprolactinemia is found, magnetic resonance imaging (MRI) with gadolinium enhancement should be performed to evaluate the pituitary fossa. A serum prolactin level greater than 200 ng/mL is strongly suggestive of pituitary adenoma.

Other recommended testing is as follows:

Measurement of follicle-stimulating hormone (FSH), luteinizing hormone (LH), and dehydroepiandrosterone sulfate (DHEAS) levels	To evaluate for hyperandrogenism when it is suggested by history and physical examination
Measurement of blood urea nitrogen (BUN) and creatinine levels	When chronic renal failure is suggested by history and physical examination
MRI of brain with gadolinium	When intracranial mass is suggested by history and physical examination

FURTHER READING

Benjamin F: Normal lactation and galactorrhea. Clin Obstet Gynecol 1994;37:887-897.

Falkenberry SS: Nipple discharge. Obstet Gynecol Clin 2002;29:21-29.

Jardines L: Management of nipple discharge. Am Surg 1996;62:119-122.

Leung AKC, Pacaud D: Diagnosis and management of galactorrhea. Am Fam Physician 2004;70:543-550.

Luciano AA: Clinical presentation of hyperprolactinemia. J Reprod Med 1999;44(12 Suppl):1085-1090.

Serri O, Chik CL, Ur E, et al: Diagnosis and management of hyperprolactinemia. CMAJ 2003;169:575-581.

Spack NP, Neinstein LS: Galactorrhea. In Neinstein LS, ed: Adolescent Health Care: A Practical Guide, 4th ed. Philadelphia: Lippincott Williams & Wilkins, 2002:1045-1051.

15 HAIR LOSS

Theodore O'Connell

Hair loss, or alopecia, can be classified in various ways, but the most common classification distinguishes nonscarring from scarring alopecia. The hair loss of scarring alopecia is permanent, whereas that of nonscarring alopecia usually is reversible. When a patient presents with hair loss, it is important to determine whether he or she is experiencing hair shedding, which is significant amounts of hair coming out, or hair thinning, in which more scalp is visible without noticeable amounts of hair falling out.

Every hair follicle goes through three phases: anagen (growth), catagen (transition between growth and resting), and telogen (resting). At any given time, approximately 85% of scalp follicles are in the anagen phase, and follicles remain in this phase for an average of 3 years. The catagen phase affects 2% to 3% of hair follicles at a time. The telogen phase occurs last, during which 10% to 15% of hair follicles undergo a rest period of about 3 months. At the end of telogen, the dead hair is ejected from the skin, and the cycle is repeated.

Alopecia areata is patchy hair loss of autoimmune origin. It usually occurs in well-circumscribed patches, but it also may involve the entire scalp (alopecia totalis) or body (alopecia universalis). The involved scalp may be normal, or subtle erythema or edema may be present. Short hairs that taper closer to the scalp surface, known as *exclamation-mark hairs*, are characteristic of alopecia areata. Alopecia areata may be associated with thyroid disease, vitiligo, or atopy. If a patient does not have any of these medical conditions and is otherwise healthy, no laboratory tests are necessary.

Androgenic alopecia, the most common form of alopecia in men and women, is also known as *male-pattern balding, female-pattern balding*, and *common balding*. Most patients with androgenic alopecia complain of thinning hair rather than shedding of hair. In some women, androgenetic alopecia may be a manifestation of hyperandrogenism; therefore, the history should focus on related signs such as menstrual irregularities, infertility, hirsutism, and acne. In an otherwise healthy woman with slowly progressive androgenetic alopecia and no signs or symptoms of hyperandrogenism, no laboratory testing is required.

Cicatricial alopecia results from a condition that damages the scalp and hair follicle. Examination typically reveals plaques of erythema with or without scaling. Syphilis, tuberculosis, acquired immunodeficiency syndrome (AIDS), herpes zoster, discoid lupus erythematosus, sarcoidosis, radiation therapy, and scalp trauma such as burns have been linked to cicatricial alopecia. If the cause of the disorder is not apparent, a punch biopsy of the scalp may be helpful in making the diagnosis.

Scarring alopecia represents a heterogeneous group of diseases manifested by erythematous papules, pustules, or scaling around hair follicles, resulting in eventual obliteration of follicular orifices.

Senescent (senile) alopecia is the steady decrease in the density of scalp hair that occurs in all persons as they age. Patients note a slow, steady, diffuse pattern of thinning hair beginning about age 50 years.

Syphilitic alopecia should be considered in every patient with unexplained hair loss. Hair loss may be rapid or slow and insidious and may be patchy (moth-eaten in appearance) or diffuse. Syphilitic alopecia is noninflammatory, nonscarring alopecia without erythema, scaling, or induration. However, in symptomatic syphilitic alopecia, the patchy or diffuse alopecia is associated with the papulosquamous lesions of secondary syphilis on the scalp or elsewhere.

Telogen effluvium occurs when an abnormally high percentage of normal hairs from all areas of the scalp enter telogen, the resting phase of hair growth. Many factors can precipitate telogen effluvium, especially stress. This disorder also may develop because of normal physiologic events such as the postpartum state or because of medications or endocrinopathies. Telogen effluvium usually begins 2 to 6 months after the causative event and lasts for several months. Hair loss is diffuse and may also affect pubic and axillary hair. Telogen effluvium is noninflammatory, and the scalp surface appears normal. The hair pull test yields positive results, although the telogen count usually does not exceed 50%.

Tinea capitis is a common condition caused by dermatophytes. Tinea capitis manifests with one or several patches of alopecia, as well as scalp inflammation. Broken-off hair shafts may create a black-dot appearance on the scalp. Fungal organisms can be displayed in a potassium hydroxide (KOH) preparation or may be cultured after adequate scraping of hair stubs from the periphery of the lesion.

Traction alopecia is a form of traumatic alopecia linked to certain methods of hair styling, including braiding, use of tight curlers, and ponytails. The outermost hairs are subjected to the most tension, and a zone of alopecia develops between braids and along the margin of the scalp.

Trichotillomania is a psychiatric impulse-control disorder in which the patient plucks the hairs. The pattern of hair loss is often suggestive of the diagnosis. One or more well-circumscribed areas of hair loss may be present, often in a bizarre pattern with incomplete areas of clearing. The scalp may be normal, or there may be areas of erythema or pustule formation. Laboratory testing is not required, but psychiatric consultation may be considered.

Medications Associated with Hair Loss

Anticonvulsants

Antithyroid agents

Chemotherapy agents

Etretinate

Heparin

Hormones

Causes of Hair Loss

Alopecia areata

Androgenetic alopecia

Scarring (cicatricial) alopecia

- AIDS
- Discoid lupus erythematosus of the scalp
- Dissecting cellulitis
- Folliculitis decalvans
- Herpes zoster
- Lichen planus follicularis (lichen planopilaris)
- Pseudopelade
- Radiation therapy
- Sarcoidosis
- Scalp trauma (burns, injuries)
- Syphilis
- Tuberculosis

Senescent (senile) alopecia

Syphilitic alopecia

Telogen effluvium

✓ Drugs

✓ Early stages of androgenetic alopecia

✓ Heavy metals

✓ High fever

✓ Hypothyroidism

✓ Major surgery

✓ Medications

✓ Postpartum effluvium

✓ Severe chronic illness

✓ Severely restrictive diets (crash or liquid protein diets)

✓ Severe infection

✓ Severe psychologic stress

Tinea capitis

Traction alopecia

Traumatic alopecia and cosmetic alopecia

Trichotillomania

Key Historical Features

✓   Shedding versus thinning

✓   Duration of the problem

✓   Broken hair versus hair shed at the roots

✓   Grooming practices (chemical treatments such as relaxers, bleaching, coloring, or blow-drying on high heat)

✓   Diet

✓   Physical or emotional stressors within the previous 3 to 6 months

✓   Medical history

✓   Medications

✓   Family history of hair loss, including hair loss in maternal relatives, paternal relatives, siblings, and children

✓   Menstrual irregularities, infertility, hirsutism, or acne in women suspected of having hyperandrogenism

Key Physical Findings

✓   Assessment of pattern of hair loss (patterned vs. diffuse hair loss)

✓   Examination of the scalp for erythema, scaling, pustules, edema, bogginess, sinus tract formation, or obliteration of follicular openings

✓   Examination of the hair shaft for caliber, shape, length, and fragility

✓   Thyroid examination

✓   Pubic or axillary hair loss

✓   Evidence of hirsutism

Suggested Work-Up

Hair pull test   Fifty to 60 hairs are grasped between the thumb and the index and middle fingers and then gently but firmly pulled. A negative test result is six or fewer hairs obtained. A positive result is more than six hairs obtained and indicates a process of active hair shedding. Microscopic evaluation of the hairs may be performed. The hair pull test is helpful in suspected cases of telogen effluvium, tinea capitis, systemic diseases, alopecia areata, alopecia totalis, alopecia universalis, and environmental factors.

Serologic test for syphilis	Recommended for all patients with unexplained hair loss to rule out syphilis

Additional Work-Up

KOH preparation for fungal elements or fungal culture of skin	In patchy forms of alopecia, to rule out fungal infection
Total testosterone, free testosterone, dehydroepiandrosterone sulfate, and prolactin level measurements	In women suspected of having hyperandrogenism
Thyroid-stimulating hormone (TSH) measurement, rapid plasma reagin (RPR) test, prolactin measurement, complete blood cell count (CBC), chemistry profile, measurement of erythrocyte sedimentation rate (ESR), antinuclear antibody (ANA) measurement, rheumatoid factor measurement, and hair pluck test for telogen:anagen ratio	In patients with telogen effluvium
CBC, ESR measurement, ANA measurement, rheumatoid factor measurement	In patients with alopecia areata
KOH examination or culture swab	In suspected cases of tinea capitis
Scalp biopsy	If the cause is unclear or if the patient fails to improve after appropriate treatment

FURTHER READING

Sperling LC, Mezebish DS: Hair diseases. Med Clin North Am 1998;82:1155-1169.

Springer K, Brown M, Stulberg DL: Common hair loss disorders. Am Fam Physician 2003;68:93-102.

Thiedke CC: Alopecia in women. Am Fam Physician 2003;67:1007-1014.

16 HEADACHE

Kathleen Dor

The majority of patients with headache experience migraine, tension-type, or medication rebound headaches. Serious or anatomic causes of headaches are uncommon but have to be considered when a patient presents with a severe headache. Headaches, particularly migraines, occur more frequently in women and can be disabling.

Migraine headaches are usually unilateral and throbbing, worsen with exercise, and typically last 4 to 72 hours. They are often accompanied by nausea, vomiting, and sensitivity to light and sound. Associated auras are usually visual or sensory disturbances. Most severe, recurrent headaches are migraines.

Tension headaches, in contrast, are usually mild and frequently can be treated with over-the-counter pain medications. Unlike migraines, they are usually bilateral and not affected by physical activity. They are often described as a pressure, ache, tightness, or "bandlike constriction" sensation around the head. Location of symptoms is commonly cervical, occipital, or temporal, although numerous variants exist. Nausea with or without vomiting may be associated with tension headaches.

Medication rebound headache should be part of the differential diagnosis for any patient with chronic daily headaches. A patient's condition may begin as migraine or tension-type headache on an episodic basis and then transform to medication rebound headache with the frequent use of analgesics. Medication rebound headache may be caused by either over-the-counter or prescription medications. Combination medications such as caffeine, aspirin, and acetaminophen (Excedrin) are often implicated.

Other types of headaches that are more common in women include trigeminal neuralgia and idiopathic intracranial hypertension (IIH) (also known as pseudotumor cerebri or benign intracranial hypertension). Trigeminal neuralgia occurs in the distribution of the trigeminal nerve, lasts only seconds to minutes, and feels like electric shocks. Headaches caused by trigeminal neuralgia can be triggered by touching the affected area. IIH is associated with papilledema and visual changes and can lead to blindness. Young obese women are at particular risk for IIH.

In evaluating a patient with a headache, it is essential to rule out a serious cause of headache by assessing any ominous findings in the history and physical examination. These findings include neurologic symptoms or signs, older age at onset, systemic illness or symptoms (such as fever, cancer, pregnancy or postpartum status, and use of anticoagulants), sudden onset of headache, new type of headache, different or progressive headache, headache that awakens the patient from sleep, and occipital headache. Headaches that can have severe consequences if they remain undiagnosed include those associated with subarachnoid hemorrhage (sudden onset) and other intracranial bleeds, IIH, meningitis (associated with fever and neck rigidity) and other infections, brain neoplasm (which may be associated with seizures), and giant cell arteritis (associated with temporal artery tenderness, diminished temporal artery pulse, jaw claudication, polymyalgia rheumatica, and visual changes).

Potential indicators of intracranial disease in patients with sudden-onset acute headache are occipitonuchal location, age of more than 40 years, and abnormal findings of neurologic examination. Symptoms of particular concern in patients with nonacute headache include increasing frequency or progressive symptoms, neurologic signs or symptoms, or pain that awakens the patient from sleep (not explained by cluster headache or typical migraine).

Medications Linked to Headache

Cimetidine

Dextroamphetamine

Diclofenac

Dipyridamole

Estrogen

Famotidine

Griseofulvin

Hydralazine

Isosorbide

Lansoprazole

Levodopa

Methylphenidate

Minoxidil

Monosodium glutamate

Nalidixic acid

Niacin

Nifedipine

Nitrites

Nitroglycerin

Omeprazole

Phenothiazines

Piroxicam

Progesterone

Pseudoephedrine

Ranitidine

Reserpine

Selective serotonin reuptake inhibitors

Sulfates

Sulfonamides

Tamoxifen

Tetracyclines

Theophylline

Trimethoprim

Tyramine

Vitamin A

Types of Headache

Cluster headache

Coital headache

Exercise-induced headache

Medication rebound headache

Migraine headache

Post—epidural injection headache

Post-traumatic headache

Tension headache

Causes of Headache

Acute angle-closure glaucoma

Arteriovenous malformation

Brain abscess

Brain tumor

Carbon monoxide exposure

Carotid artery dissection

Cerebral venous thrombosis

Cervical spondylosis

Chronic paroxysmal hemicrania

Encephalitis

Generalized seizure

Giant cell arteritis (temporal arteritis)

Granulomatous angiitis

Human immunodeficiency virus (HIV) infection

Hydrocephalus

Hypercapnia caused by chronic obstructive lung disease

Hypertension encephalopathy

Hyperthyroidism

Hypothyroidism

IIH (Idiopathic intracranial hypertension)

Intracerebral hemorrhage

Ischemic stroke

Meningitis

Polyarteritis nodosa (vasculitis)

Preeclampsia

Rheumatoid arthritis (vasculitis)

Sinusitis

Sleep apnea

Subarachnoid hemorrhage

Systemic lupus erythematosus (vasculitis)

Temporomandibular joint (TMJ) syndrome

Trigeminal neuralgia

Key Historical Features

✓   Location of headache

✓   Nature of headache

✓   Pattern of headache

✓   Duration of headache

✓   Frequency of headache

✓   Severity of headache

✓   Age when headaches first experienced

✓   Triggers (exercise, food, sex, coughing, cold liquids)

✓   Associated symptoms

- Fever

- Nausea or vomiting

- Stiff neck

- • Neck pain
- • Vision changes
- • Rash
- • Nasal congestion
- • Facial pain
- • Jaw claudication
- • Myalgias

✓ Auras

✓ Recent lumbar puncture/epidural injection

✓ Recent trauma

✓ Medical history, especially that of the following:

- • Prior headaches
- • Cancer
- • Lung disease
- • HIV infection
- • Thyroid disease
- • Hypertension
- • Stroke
- • Preeclampsia
- • Heart disease

✓ Surgical history

✓ Obstetric history

✓ Social history

- • Tobacco, alcohol, drugs, caffeine use
- • Diet and physical activity
- • Domestic violence

✓ Family history, especially of headaches

✓ Medications, including anticoagulants and pain medications

✓ Neurologic symptoms

- • Change in mental status
- • Memory loss
- • Personality changes
- • Numbness
- • Weakness
- • Balance problems

- Speech difficulty
- Loss of consciousness
- Dizziness
- Tinnitus
- Seizures

✓ Psychologic symptoms

- Stressors
- Sleep history and whether headaches awaken patient from sleep
- History or symptoms of depression, anxiety, or personality disorders

✓ Gynecologic/obstetric symptoms

- Relation of headache to menstrual cycle
- Date of most recent menstrual period

✓ Gastrointestinal symptoms

- Right upper quadrant abdominal pain, which may be associated with preeclampsia

Key Physical Findings

✓ Vital signs, especially hypertension or fever

✓ Body mass index

✓ General assessment of well-being and mental status

✓ Head and neck examination for evidence of ear infection; sinusitis; TMJ syndrome; neck stiffness; neck tenderness; or temporal artery tenderness, swelling, or erythema

✓ Funduscopic examination to evaluate for papilledema

✓ Neurologic examination (complete)

✓ Musculoskeletal examination for any muscle tenderness or trigger points

Suggested Work-Up

In the absence of neurologic findings, episodic migraine does not necessitate imaging studies. The evidence is less clear for chronic headache, whether migraine or nonmigraine.

The American Academy of Neurology states that neuroimaging should be considered in patients with unexplained abnormal findings on the neurologic examination, but it also states that there is no clear evidence to recommend magnetic resonance imaging (MRI) or computed tomographic (CT) scanning as the initial examination.

Patients who have had a stable headache pattern for at least 6 months rarely have significant intracranial disease. In the absence of worrisome features, these patients do not require imaging.

Features that raise the index of suspicion for a pathologic cause in patients with chronic or recurrent headaches include systemic symptoms or illness (especially fever, change in mentation, use of anticoagulation, current or recent pregnancy, or cancer), neurologic symptoms or signs (papilledema, asymmetric cranial nerve or motor function, or abnormal cerebellar function), recent or sudden onset of headache, onset after 40 years of age, or history of a different type of headache or progression of severity of headaches.

If there are features that raise the index of suspicion for a pathologic cause, as mentioned previously, brain MRI or brain CT scanning should be performed.

Additional Work-Up

Complete blood cell count	If infection or anemia is suspected
HIV test	If the patient is at risk for HIV infection
Lumbar puncture	If meningitis or subarachnoid hemorrhage is suspected
Blood culture	If meningitis is suspected
Measurement of erythrocyte sedimentation rate	If giant cell arteritis is suspected
Temporal artery biopsy	If giant cell arteritis is suspected
Thyroid-stimulating hormone (TSH)	If thyroid disease is suspected
Urine pregnancy test	If pregnancy is suspected
Urinalysis	To evaluate for proteinuria in a pregnant patient
Liver function tests and measurement of creatinine, uric acid, and lactate dehydrogenase	If preeclampsia is suspected

Measurement of prothrombin time, partial prothrombin time, and international normalized ratio (INR)	If preeclampsia or hemorrhage is suspected or a patient is taking an anticoagulant
Sinus radiography or CT scanning	If sinusitis is suspected

FURTHER READING

Dodick DW: Clinical clues and clinical rules: primary vs secondary headache. Adv Stud Med 2003;3:S550-S555.

Frishberg BM: The utility of neuroimaging in the evaluation of headache in patients with normal neurologic examinations. Neurology 1994;44:1191-1197.

Johnson CJ: Headache in women. Prim Care 2004;31:417-428.

Levin M: The many causes of headache: migraine, vascular, drug-induced, and more. Postgrad Medicine 2002;112(6):67-6871-72, 75-76.

Maizels M: The patient with daily headaches. Am Fam Physician 2004;70:2299-2306.

Marcus DA: Focus on primary care: diagnosis and management of headache in women. Obstet Gynecol Surv 1999;54:395-402.

Paulson GW: Headaches in women, including women who are pregnant. Am J Obstet Gynecol 1995;173;1734-1741.

Silberstein SD: Practice parameter: evidence-based guidelines for migraine headache (an evidence-based review): report of the Quality Standards Subcommittee of the American Academy of Neurology. Neurology 2000;55:754-762.

Theodore O'Connell

Definitions of microscopic hematuria vary from 1 to more than 10 red blood cells per high-power field on microscopic evaluation of urinary sediment from two of three properly collected urinalysis specimens. The American Urological Association has issued guidelines (Figs. 17-1 and 17-2) for the evaluation of microscopic hematuria in adults and defines clinically significant microscopic hematuria as three or more red blood cells per high-power field. However, each laboratory establishes its own thresholds on the basis of the method of detection used.

Dipstick testing for heme lacks specificity, inasmuch as the presence of myoglobin or hemoglobin may result in a positive test result when the urine contains no red blood cells. If the dipstick test is positive, the presence of red blood cells should be confirmed by microscopic examination of the urine. If the urine dipstick test reveals blood, as well as leukocyte esterase, nitrites, and bacteria consistent with urinary tract infection, treatment with antibiotics is appropriate. If the hematuria resolves with treatment, no additional evaluation is necessary, but serum creatinine should be measured.

Microscopic hematuria may be transient, caused by vigorous exercise, mild trauma, sexual intercourse, or by menstrual contamination. If transient microscopic hematuria is suspected, urinalysis should be repeated 48 hours after discontinuation of these activities. Persistent microscopic hematuria warrants further evaluation.

Causes of microscopic hematuria may be classified as either glomerular or nonglomerular in origin. Immunoglobulin A nephropathy is the most common glomerular cause. Nonglomerular causes involving the kidney and upper urinary tract include nephrolithiasis, neoplasm, polycystic kidney disease, medullary sponge kidney, papillary necrosis, hypercalciuria, and hyperuricosuria. Causes involving the lower urinary tract include disorders of the bladder or urethra, such as bladder cancer.

The urinalysis is the most important test in the evaluation of hematuria because it often distinguishes glomerular from nonglomerular bleeding. If proteinuria is detected on dipstick testing, total urinary protein excretion should be quantified. Twenty-four-hour urinary protein excretion of more than 300 mg suggests the kidney as a source of microscopic hematuria. Other findings that support a glomerular cause include renal insufficiency, red blood cell casts, or dysmorphic red blood cells. When glomerular bleeding is suggested, no urologic evaluation is necessary. Proteinuria or renal insufficiency with microscopic hematuria warrants referral to a nephrologist for evaluation and possible renal biopsy.

If a glomerular source is ruled out or considered unlikely, the upper urinary tract should undergo imaging. Excretory urography, ultrasonography, computed tomographic (CT) scanning, or magnetic resonance imaging (MRI) may be used. A CT scan without contrast medium is appropriate as the first test for patients with suspected urinary stone disease. When there is no clinical suspicion of urinary stone disease, CT urography should be performed, first without and then with contrast medium. CT scanning is more expensive than excretory urography and ultrasonography, but it is the best imaging modality for the evaluation of urinary stones, renal and perirenal infections, and associated complications. In addition, with excretory urography and ultrasonography, additional imaging is often necessary for further evaluating cysts. When CT scanning is unavailable, excretory urography or ultrasonography are reasonable alternatives individually or in combination. Ultrasonography is advised in place of CT scanning for patients with renal failure, pregnancy, or hypersensitivity to contrast medium.

The source of microscopic hematuria is not found in about 70% of cases after urinalysis for evidence of glomerular hematuria and imaging of the upper urinary tract. The work-up usually proceeds with evaluation of the lower urinary tract. Cystoscopy is appropriate if risk factors for bladder cancer are present. Cytologic analysis of voided urine is less sensitive than cystoscopy in the detection of bladder cancer, but it has high specificity. The sensitivity is improved if specimens of urine are obtained from the first voiding in the morning on 3 consecutive days.

Patients at risk for significant disease include those with a history of smoking or analgesic abuse; those with occupational exposure to benzenes or aromatic amines; those older than 40 years; those with a history of gross hematuria, urologic disease, irritative voiding symptoms, or urinary tract infection; and those with a history of pelvic irradiation.

A thorough evaluation of the urinary system may fail to identify a source of microscopic hematuria in 19% to 68% of patients. In patients with a negative initial finding in evaluation of asymptomatic microscopic hematuria, the clinician should consider repeating urinalysis, voided urine cytologic testing, and blood pressure determination at 6, 12, 24, and 36 months. Additional evaluation, including repeated imaging and cystoscopy, may be warranted in patients with persistent hematuria in whom significant underlying disease is strongly suspected. If gross hematuria, abnormal urinary cytologic findings, or irritative voiding symptoms in the absence of infection develop, reevaluation should be undertaken immediately. This may include cystoscopy, urinary cytologic testing, or repeated imaging.

Medications Linked to Hematuria

Aminoglycosides

Amitriptyline

Anticonvulsants

Aspirin

Busulfan

Captopril

Cephalosporins

Chlorpromazine

Ciprofloxacin

Cyclophosphamide

Diuretics

Furosemide

Heparin

Indinavir

Mirtazapine

Nonsteroidal anti-inflammatory
drugs (NSAIDs)

Omeprazole

Oral contraceptives

Penicillins

Quinine

Rifampin

Ritonavir

Triamterene

Trimethoprim-sulfamethoxazole

Vincristine

Warfarin

Causes of Microscopic Hematuria

Glomerular Causes

- Immunoglobulin A nephropathy
- Fabry disease
- Goodpasture syndrome
- Hemolytic uremic syndrome
- Henoch-Schönlein purpura
- Hereditary nephritis (Alport syndrome)
- Lupus nephritis
- Membranoproliferative glomerulonephritis
- Mesangial proliferative glomerulonephritis
- Mild focal glomerulonephritis of other causes

- Nail-patella syndrome
- Polyarteritis
- Postinfectious glomerulonephritis (endocarditis or viral)
- Poststreptococcal glomerulonephritis
- Thin basement membrane disease
- Wegener granulomatosis

Nonglomerular Causes

Upper urinary tract causes

- Cytomegalovirus
- Epstein-Barr virus infection
- Hereditary nephritis
- Hypercalciuria
- Hyperuricosuria
- Loin pain—hematuria syndrome
- Lymphoma
- Malignant hypertension
- Medications
- Medullary sponge kidney
- Multicystic kidney disease
- Nephrolithiasis
- Papillary necrosis
- Polycystic kidney disease
- Pyelonephritis
- Renal arteriovenous malformation
- Renal cell carcinoma
- Renal infarction
- Renal venous thrombosis
- Renal trauma
- Renal tuberculosis
- Sarcoidosis
- Schistosomiasis
- Sickle cell trait or disease
- Sjögren syndrome
- Solitary renal cyst
- Syphilis
- Toxoplasmosis
- Tuberculosis

- Ureteral stricture
- Ureteral transitional-cell carcinoma

Lower urinary tract causes

- Benign bladder polyps and tumors
- Benign ureteral polyps and tumors
- Bladder cancer
- Calculi
- Coagulopathy
- Congenital abnormalities
- Cystitis
- Endometriosis
- Epididymitis
- Foreign bodies
- Perineal irritation
- Posterior ureteral valves
- Radiation-induced inflammation
- Schistosomiasis
- Transitional cell carcinoma of ureter or bladder
- Trauma (catheterization, blunt trauma)
- Urethral and meatal strictures
- Urethritis

Other causes

- Benign hematuria
- Exercise hematuria
- Factitious hematuria
- Menstrual contamination
- Over-anticoagulation with warfarin
- Sexual intercourse

Key Historical Features

✓ Irritative voiding

✓ Medical history, especially history of urologic disease or pelvic irradiation

✓ Medications

✓ Cigarette smoking

✓ Travel history

✓ Occupational exposure to benzene or aromatic amines

Key Physical Findings

✓ Vital signs, especially blood pressure measurement

✓ General examination

✓ Cardiac examination for irregular rhythm, suggestive of atrial fibrillation, or new murmur, suggestive of endocarditis

✓ Abdominal examination for bruits, masses, organomegaly, or aortic aneurysm

✓ Back examination for costovertebral angle tenderness

✓ Urethral and vaginal examination

✓ Extremity examination for peripheral edema or petechiae

Suggested Work-Up

Urinalysis	To evaluate for bacteriuria and pyuria
Urine culture	Should be obtained if the urinalysis reveals bacteriuria or pyuria
Serum creatinine	To evaluate for renal insufficiency
CT urography without and with contrast medium (excretory urography and ultrasonography are alternatives when CT scanning is unavailable or too expensive); ultrasonography is advised in place of CT scanning for patients with renal failure, pregnancy, or hypersensitivity to contrast medium	To evaluate the upper urinary tract for renal-cell carcinoma, transitional cell carcinomas, urolithiasis, cystic disease, and obstructive lesions
Cytologic analysis of urine (first void in the morning on 3 consecutive days)	To evaluate for bladder cancer and carcinoma in situ
Cystoscopy	Recommended for all persons with asymptomatic microscopic hematuria who are older than 40 years and for those who are younger but have risk factors for bladder cancer

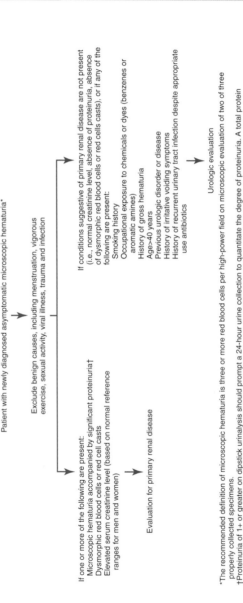

Figure 17-1. Initial evaluation of newly diagnosed microscopic hematuria. (Adapted from Grossfeld GD, Wolf JS, Litwin MS, et al: Asymptomatic microscopic hematuria in adults: summary of the AUA best practice policy recommendations. Am Fam Physician 2001;63:1145-1154, Figures 1 and 2.)

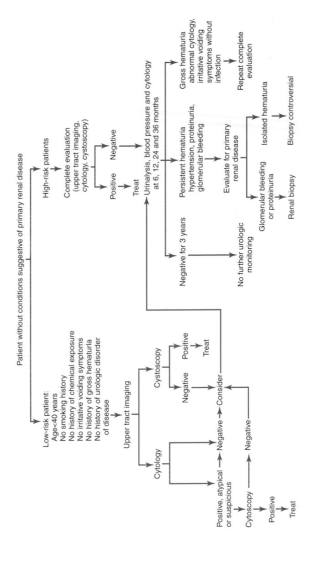

Figure 17-2. Urologic evaluation of asymptomatic microscopic hematuria.

Additional Work-Up

Measurement of the ratio of urinary protein to urinary creatinine concentration *or* 24-hour urine collection is recommended if proteinuria is detected on dipstick testing to determine total protein excretion.

FURTHER READING

Ahmed Z, Lee J: Hematuria and proteinuria. Med Clin North Am 1997;81:641-652.

Cohen RA, Brown RS: Microscopic hematuria. N Engl J Med 2003;348:2330-2338.

Feld LG, Waz WR, Perez LM, et al: Hematuria. An integrated medical and surgical approach. Pediatr Clin North Am 1997;44:1191-1210.

Grossfeld GD, Carroll PR: Evaluation of asymptomatic microscopic hematuria. Urol Clin North Am 1998;25:661-676.

Grossfeld GD, Wolf JS, Litwin MS, et al: Asymptomatic microscopic hematuria in adults: summary of the AUA best practice policy recommendations. Am Fam Physician 2001;63: 1145-1154.

Harper M, Arya M, Hamid R, et al: Haematuria: a streamlined approach to management. Hosp Med 2001;62:696-698.

Mazhari R, Kimmel PL: Hematuria: an algorithmic approach to finding the cause. Cleve Clin J Med 2002;69:870-876.

McDonald MM, Swagerty D: Assessment of microscopic hematuria in adults. Am Fam Physician 2006;73:1748-1754.

Sokolosky MC: Hematuria. Emerg Med Clin North Am 2001;19:621-632.

Thaller TR, Wang LP: Evaluation of asymptomatic microscopic hematuria in adults. Am Fam Physician 1999;60:1143-1154.

Yun EJ, Meng MV, Carroll PR: Evaluation of the patient with hematuria. Med Clin North Am 2004;88:329-343.

18 HIRSUTISM

Theodore O'Connell

Hirsutism is defined as the presence of excessive coarse terminal hair in a pattern not normal in women in areas such as the face, chest, or upper abdomen. This disorder is a sign of increased androgen action on hair follicles, which may result from increased levels of endogenous or exogenous androgens or from increased sensitivity of hair follicles to normal levels of circulating androgens.

In evaluating hirsutism, it is important to determine whether hirsutism exists alone or whether virilization is also present. This distinction is important because virilization may reflect a serious underlying pathologic condition, such as malignancy. Virilization manifests with a wide range of signs of androgen excess in addition to hirsutism, such as acne, frontotemporal balding, amenorrhea, oligomenorrhea, deepening of the voice, and clitoromegaly.

The most common triggering mechanism for hirsutism is excess androgen production. Although androgens may come from an exogenous source, androgen excess is most commonly endogenous. The two primary sources of endogenous androgens are the adrenal glands and the ovaries. Adrenal gland—related causes include congenital adrenal hyperplasia, Cushing syndrome, or tumor. Ovarian causes include polycystic ovary syndrome and tumors.

Medications Linked to Hirsutism

Anabolic steroids

Danazol

Methyldopa

Metoclopramide

Phenothiazines

Progestins (especially levonorgestrel, norethindrone, and norgestrel)

Reserpine

Testosterone

Causes of Hirsutism

Congenital adrenal hyperplasia

Cushing syndrome

Exogenous pharmacologic source of androgens

Familial hirsutism

Idiopathic

Medications

Polycystic ovary syndrome

Tumor (ovarian, adrenal, or pituitary)

Key Historical Features

✓ Onset and extent of hair growth

✓ Medical history

✓ Menstrual and reproductive history

✓ Medications

✓ Family history

✓ Weight gain

✓ Abdominal symptoms

✓ Breast discharge or galactorrhea

✓ Skin signs such as acne, dryness, or striae

✓ Signs of virilization

Key Physical Findings

✓ Blood pressure, height, weight

✓ Evaluation of hair distribution and characteristics

✓ Skin evaluation (for acanthosis nigricans, acne, striae, hyperpigmentation)

✓ Breast examination for nipple discharge or galactorrhea

✓ Abdominal examination for masses

✓ Pelvic examination for masses

✓ Signs of Cushing syndrome

✓ Signs of virilization

Suggested Work-Up

Measurement of serum testosterone, serum 17α-hydroxyprogesterone, and dehydroepiandrosterone sulfate (DHEAS)	To evaluate for ovarian and adrenal tumors and adult-onset adrenal hyperplasia

Serum prolactin measurement	To evaluate for pituitary tumors
Thyroid-stimulating hormone (TSH) measurement	To evaluate for thyroid dysfunction
Fasting serum glucose measurement	To evaluate for insulin resistance in patients suspected of having polycystic ovary syndrome

Additional Work-Up

Adrenocorticotropic hormone (ACTH) stimulation test	When Cushing syndrome or adult-onset congenital adrenal hyperplasia is suspected
Glucose tolerance test	In patients with suspected polycystic ovary syndrome with elevated fasting serum glucose levels
CT scanning of the abdomen and pelvis	To assess the adrenal glands and ovaries in patients whose history, physical examination findings, or laboratory evaluation results are suggestive of the presence of a virilizing tumor

FURTHER READING

Gilchrist VJ, Hecht BR: A practical approach to hirsutism. Am Fam Physician 1995;52:1837-1846.

Hunter MH, Carek PJ: Evaluation and treatment of women with hirsutism. Am Fam Physician 2003;67:2565-2572.

Leung AK, Robson WL: Hirsutism. Int J Dermatol 1993;32:773-777.

Plouffe L: Disorders of excessive hair growth in the adolescent. Obstet Gynecol Clin 2000;27:79-99.

Redmond GP, Bergfeld WF: Diagnostic approach to androgen disorders in women: acne, hirsutism, and alopecia. Cleve Clin J Med 1990;57:423-427.

Speroff L, Glass RH, Kase NG, eds: Clinical Gynecologic Endocrinology and Infertility, 6th ed. Baltimore: Lippincott Williams & Wilkins, 1999:529-556.

Kathleen Dor

Hypertension is defined as systolic blood pressure of 140 or higher, a diastolic blood pressure of 90 or higher, or both. Women with hypertension during pregnancy need to be monitored carefully because of the significant risk of morbidity and mortality in the mother, fetus, and newborn. Hypertension during pregnancy is classified as gestational hypertension, preeclampsia, eclampsia, or chronic hypertension.

Gestational hypertension is hypertension that develops after 20 weeks of pregnancy and resolves by 12 weeks post partum. About 25% of women with gestational hypertension develop preeclampsia. Preeclampsia is gestational hypertension that is associated with proteinuria (≥ 0.3 g of protein/24 hours). Eclampsia is the presence of seizures in a pregnant woman with preeclampsia.

Risk factors for preeclampsia include first pregnancy, multiple fetuses, chronic hypertension, diabetes, renal disease, thrombophilia, vascular and connective tissue disease, obesity, maternal age of greater than 35 years, or maternal age of less than 20 years.

Chronic hypertension is hypertension that starts before the 20th week of pregnancy. Patients with chronic hypertension are at considerable risk of developing superimposed preeclampsia. Possible complications of chronic hypertension include preterm labor, intrauterine growth restriction, fetal death, and placental abruption.

Medications and Supplements Associated with Hypertension during Pregnancy

Bitter orange

Cyclooxygenase-2 (COX-2) inhibitors

Cyclosporine

Ephedra

Erythropoietin

Ma huang

Nonsteroidal anti-inflammatory drugs (NSAIDs)

Oral contraceptives

Steroids

Sympathomimetic drugs

- Anorectics
- Decongestants

Tacrolimus

Causes of Hypertension During Pregnancy

Alcohol intake

Chronic hypertension

Coarctation of the aorta

Cushing syndrome

Essential hypertension

Pheochromocytoma

Primary aldosteronism

Renal artery disease

Renal disease

Sleep apnea

Thyroid disease

Chronic hypertension with superimposed preeclampsia or eclampsia

Diet (licorice)

Eclampsia

Gestational hypertension

Illicit drug use

- Amphetamines
- Cocaine

Medications

Obesity

Preeclampsia

- Mild preeclampsia
- Severe preeclampsia

Key Historical Features

✓ Obstetric history

- Gravity and parity
- Previous obstetric complications, including hypertension, diabetes, fetal loss, preterm labor
- Gestational age or most recent menstrual period
- Fetal movement
- Contractions
- Vaginal bleeding
- Rupture of membranes

✓ Medical history, especially history of the following:

- Diabetes mellitus
- Hypertension

- Vascular and connective tissue disease
- Kidney disease
- Thrombophilia
- Thyroid disease

✓ Medications

✓ Social history

- Tobacco, alcohol, or illicit drug use

✓ Family history, especially history of hypertension, kidney disease, or diabetes

✓ Neurologic symptoms

- Headaches and visual disturbances, which are associated with severe preeclampsia

✓ Gastrointestinal symptoms

- Epigastric and/or right upper quadrant pain, both of which are associated with severe preeclampsia

✓ Renal

- Oliguria, which may be associated with severe preeclampsia

Key Physical Findings

✓ Vital signs

- Blood pressure should be measured with the patient either sitting up or in the left lateral recumbent position; the patient's arm should be at the level of the heart; patients should be seated for at least 5 minutes before the measurement, and at least two measurements should be made; and an appropriate size cuff should be used (cuff bladder encircles at least 80% of the arm)

✓ General evaluation for rapid weight gain or facial edema, because fluid retention is associated with preeclampsia

✓ Funduscopic examination for evidence of retinopathy in patients with chronic hypertension

✓ Cardiovascular examination for arrhythmias, heart murmurs, abnormal heart sounds, carotid or femoral bruits, and peripheral pulses

✓ Pulmonary examination for evidence of pulmonary edema

✓ Obstetric evaluation to determine fundal height for fetal growth

✓ Gastrointestinal examination for right upper quadrant tenderness, liver enlargement, or an enlarged kidney

Suggested Work-Up

Urinalysis	To evaluate for proteinuria and glucosuria
Twenty-four-hour urine sampling for total protein *or* spot urine protein/creatinine ratio	To evaluate for and quantify proteinuria
Complete blood cell count	Because hemoconcentration occurs with preeclampsia and because hemolysis and thrombocytopenia may be associated with preeclampsia as part of the syndrome of hemolysis, elevated liver enzyme counts, and low platelet count (HELLP)
Serum creatinine measurement	Elevated creatinine levels may be associated with chronic kidney disease or preeclampsia

In women who develop hypertension after 20 weeks, the following testing should be performed in addition to the tests just described:

Uric acid measurement	Elevated uric acid level is associated with preeclampsia
Lactate dehydrogenase (LDH) measurement	Elevated LDH level may be a sign of hemolysis
Partial thromboplastin time (PTT), prothrombin time (PT), and international normalized ratio (INR) measurements	To evaluate for coagulopathy
Alanine transaminase (ALT) and aspartate transaminase (AST) measurements	Elevated liver enzyme levels are suggestive of severe preeclampsia

Additional Work-Up

Obstetric ultrasonography	Baseline ultrasonography should be performed at 18 to 20 weeks of pregnancy
	According to the Working Group on High Blood Pressure in Pregnancy,

	ultrasonography for fetal growth and amniotic fluid should be repeated every 3 weeks in patients with mild preeclampsia if the sonograms are normal
	In patients with chronic hypertension, ultrasonography should be repeated only if there is a change in maternal or fetal condition or if fetal growth cannot be assessed through fundal height measurement (e.g., with maternal obesity)
Nonstress test and biophysical profile	Both should be performed regularly to evaluate fetal well-being
Electrocardiography	To evaluate for evidence of left ventricular hypertrophy in patients with chronic hypertension
Echocardiography	May be considered in patients with chronic hypertension to evaluate for left ventricular hypertrophy

FURTHER READING

ACOG Committee on Practice Bulletins: ACOG Practice Bulletin. Chronic hypertension in pregnancy. ACOG Committee on Practice Bulletins. Obstet Gynecol 2001;98(1):Suppl 177-185.

ACOG Committee on Practice Bulletins—Obstetrics: ACOG practice bulletin. Diagnosis and management of preeclampsia and eclampsia. Number 33, January 2002. Obstet Gynecol 2002;99:159-167.

Beckmann CRB, Ling FW, Smith RP, et al. Hypertension in Pregnacy. In Obstetrics and Gynecology, 5th ed. Philadelphia: Lippincott Williams & Wilkins, 2006, pp. 188-196.

Report of the National High Blood Pressure Education Program Working Group on High Blood Pressure in Pregnancy. Am J Obstet Gynecol 2000;183(1):S1-S22.

The Seventh Report of the Joint National Committee on the Prevention, Detection, Evaluation and Treatment of High Blood Pressure. Washington, DC: U.S. Department of Human and Health Services, December 2003.

Wagner LK: Diagnosis and management of preeclampsia. Am Fam Physician 2004;70:2317-2324.

Zamorski MA, Green LA: NHBPEP report on high blood pressure in pregnancy: a summary for family physicians. Am Fam Physician 2001;64:263-270.

Theodore O'Connell

Hyperthyroidism is a hypermetabolic state that results from excess synthesis and release of thyroid hormone, usually from the thyroid gland. The overall incidence of subclinical and overt hyperthyroidism is estimated to be 0.05% to 0.1% in the general population. Hyperthyroidism occurs in all age groups and is more common in women than in men. Graves' disease is the most common cause of hyperthyroidism, causing 60% to 80% of cases. However, toxic nodular goiter is the most common cause of hyperthyroidism in the elderly.

Hyperthyroidism may manifest as a condition in a spectrum ranging from asymptomatic, subclinical hyperthyroidism to life-threatening thyroid storm. Subclinical hyperthyroidism is diagnosed in asymptomatic patients with low levels of thyroid-stimulating hormone (TSH) but normal free thyroxine (T4) and free triiodothyronine (T3). Clinical hyperthyroidism manifests with the typical signs and symptoms outlined later in this chapter.

In elderly patients, the condition often represents a diagnostic challenge because they may have lone symptoms or atypical manifestations. They may have negative symptoms such as depression, lethargy, or apathetic facies. Elderly patients also may have only a small goiter, weight loss, worsening of underlying cardiovascular disease, or new-onset atrial fibrillation.

Medications Linked to Hyperthyroidism

Amiodarone

Alemtuzumab (Campath 1-H) (a monoclonal antibody)

Highly active antiretroviral therapy (HAART)

Interferon-α

Lithium

Causes of Hyperthyroidism

Factitious hyperthyroidism

Graves disease

Iodine-induced hyperthyroidism (iodine ingestion, radiographic contrast medium, amiodarone ingestion)

Lymphocytic thyroiditis (Hashimoto thyroiditis)

Medication-induced thyroiditis

Metastatic thyroid cancer

Ovarian tumors (struma ovarii)

Pituitary adenoma—secreting TSH

Postpartum thyroiditis

Toxic adenoma

Toxic multinodular goiter

Trophoblastic tumor

Key Historical Features

✓ Constitutional symptoms

- Anxiety
- Excessive perspiration
- Fatigue
- Heat intolerance
- Nervousness
- Pruritus
- Thirst
- Weight loss

✓ Cardiac symptoms

- Anginal symptoms
- Exertional dyspnea
- Orthopnea
- Palpitations
- Reduced exercise tolerance

✓ Pulmonary symptoms

- Dyspnea

✓ Gastrointestinal symptoms

- Difficulty swallowing
- Dyspepsia
- Frequent bowel movements
- Nausea and vomiting
- Rapid intestinal transit time

✓ Genitourinary symptoms

- Nocturia
- Urinary frequency

✓ Ophthalmologic symptoms

- Diplopia
- Eye irritation or dryness

- Excessive tearing
- Pain with eye movements
- Visual blurring

✓ Reproductive symptoms

- Amenorrhea
- Decreased libido
- Gynecomastia
- Infertility
- Menometrorrhagia
- Oligomenorrhea
- Spider angiomas

✓ Neuromuscular symptoms

- Fatigability
- Generalized weakness
- Proximal muscle weakness

✓ Psychiatric symptoms

- Altered mental status
- Emotional lability
- Insomnia
- Memory loss
- Nightmares and vivid dreams
- Poor attention span
- Restlessness

✓ Medical history

✓ Recent pregnancy

✓ Smoking

✓ Family history

Key Physical Findings

✓ Vital signs, especially signs of tachycardia or hypertension

✓ Skin and hair

- Warm, smooth, velvety skin
- Skin hyperpigmentation
- Palmar erythema
- Pretibial myxedema
- Fine, brittle scalp hair

- Diffuse alopecia
- Nail changes (onycholysis)

✓ Ocular signs

- Exophthalmos
- Proptosis
- Eyelid lag
- Infrequent blinking
- Vasodilation of the conjunctiva
- Eyelid or periorbital edema
- Papilledema

✓ Thyroid signs

- Diffuse enlargement
- Single nodule
- Multinodular goiter
- Bruit

✓ Cardiovascular signs

- Tachycardia
- Bounding pulses
- Rapid and brisk carotid upstroke
- Systolic flow murmurs
- Atrial arrhythmias such as atrial fibrillation or atrial flutter

✓ Pulmonary signs

- Tachypnea

✓ Musculoskeletal signs

- Decreased muscle strength
- Decreased muscle volume
- Muscle atrophy
- Muscle weakness, especially proximal

✓ Neurologic signs

- Brisk reflexes
- Fidgeting
- Nervousness
- Hyperactivity and rapid speech

Suggested Work-Up

TSH	To evaluate thyroid function
Radionuclide uptake scan	To distinguish Graves disease from thyroiditis and provide anatomic information

Additional Work-Up

Thyroglobulin level

May help distinguish Graves disease (elevated thyroglobulin level) from factitious thyrotoxicosis (decreased thyroglobulin level)

Measurement of thyroid peroxidase antibodies

Elevated levels in Graves disease and lymphocytic thyroiditis

FURTHER READING

Ginsberg J: Diagnosis and management of Graves' disease. CMAJ 2003;168:575-585.

McKeown NJ, Tews MC, Gossain V V, et al: Hyperthyroidism. Emerg Med Clin North Am 2005;23:669-685.

Reid JR, Wheeler SF: Hyperthyroidism: diagnosis and treatment. Am Fam Physician 2005;72:623-630.

21 HYPOTHYROIDISM

Kathleen Dor

Hypothyroidism usually results from decreased thyroid hormone production and secretion by the thyroid gland. Hypothyroidism can be either primary or central. Central hypothyroidism involves either the pituitary gland (secondary hypothyroidism) or the hypothalamus (tertiary hypothyroidism). In the United States, the most common cause of hypothyroidism is chronic autoimmune thyroiditis.

Hypothyroidism is far more common in women and in the elderly than in other populations. In fact, about 2% to 3% of older women have hypothyroidism. Other risk factors include the presence of thyroid peroxidase antibodies and a high normal level of TSH.

Untreated hypothyroidism can result in decreased cardiac output, memory loss, infertility, and sleep apnea. The American Academy of Family Physicians recommends screening for hypothyroidism in patients 60 years of age or older and in patients with symptoms of hypothyroidism, a family history of thyroid disease, a history of autoimmune disease, or type 1 diabetes.

Myxedema coma refers to severe complications of hypothyroidism, involving hypothermia and stupor or coma. Myxedema coma can be precipitated by mild illnesses, exposure to cold, myocardial infarction, and medications that affect the central nervous system.

During pregnancy, there is a greater requirement of thyroid hormone because of increased maternal use, as well as transportation of thyroid hormone across the placenta. Some women who were euthyroid before pregnancy become hypothyroid during pregnancy. It is very important that women be treated adequately for hypothyroidism during pregnancy to avoid complications such as miscarriage, preeclampsia, preterm labor, and postpartum hemorrhage.

Medications That Can Cause Hypothyroidism

Amiodarone

Ethionamide

Interferon-α

Interleukin-2

Iodine excess

Lithium

Methimazole

Propylthiouracil

Sulfonamides

Causes of Hypothyroidism

Primary Hypothyroidism

Agenesis and dysgenesis of the thyroid gland

External irradiation

Hashimoto disease (chronic autoimmune thyroiditis)

Infections

- *Mycobacterium tuberculosis*
- *Pneumocystis carinii*

Infiltrative disorders

- Amyloidosis
- Hemochromatosis
- Leukemia
- Lymphoma
- Sarcoidosis
- Scleroderma

Invasive fibrous thyroiditis

Iodine deficiency

Medications

Postpartum thyroiditis

Radioactive iodine therapy

Silent thyroiditis

Subacute thyroiditis

Thyroid hormone resistance

Thyroidectomy

Secondary/Tertiary Hypothyroidism (Central Hypothyroidism)

- Chronic lymphocytic hypophysitis
- Congenital abnormalities (defects in thyrotropin-releasing hormone, TSH, or both)
- Infections
- Infiltrative disorders
- Other brain tumors (nonpituitary)
- Pituitary tumors, metastasis, hemorrhage, necrosis, and aneurysms
- Surgery
- Trauma

Key Historical Features

✓ Associated symptoms

- Fatigue
- Weakness
- Depression
- Sleep disturbances
- Decreased appetite
- Memory loss
- Intolerance of cold
- Decreased sweating
- Weight gain
- Muscle cramps
- Dry skin
- Brittle nails
- Coarse hair
- Hair loss
- Hearing loss
- Hoarseness
- Facial swelling
- Pretibial swelling
- Menorrhagia
- Infertility
- Constipation
- Paresthesias
- Changes in senses of taste and smell

✓ Medical history, especially diseases associated with hypothyroidism, such as diabetes mellitus, hyperlipidemia, Sjögren syndrome, pernicious anemia, systemic lupus erythematous, rheumatoid arthritis, primary biliary cirrhosis, chronic hepatitis, vitiligo, and carpal tunnel syndrome

Key Physical Findings

✓ Vital signs

✓ Head and neck examination

- Thyroid nodules or goiter (note any thyroidectomy scars)
- Ophthalmopathy (proptosis, periorbital edema, conjunctival injection, abnormal extraocular muscle function), which occurs in 4% to 9% of patients with Hashimoto thyroiditis

- • Pemberton sign: facial plethora, raised jugular venous pressure, and inspiratory stridor when the patient raises arms above her head, which indicates a neck mass such as goiter
✓ Cardiovascular examination
  - • Bradycardia, associated with hypothyroidism
  - • Pericardial effusion
✓ Gastrointestinal examination for ascites
✓ Pulmonary examination for a pleural effusion
✓ Neurologic examination for proximal weakness, peripheral neuropathy, and a slow return of deep tendon reflexes

Suggested Work-Up

TSH measurement	Levels are high in primary hypothyroidism and subclinical hypothyroidism; levels are low, normal, or minimally elevated in central hypothyroidism
Free thyroxine (T4) measurement	Levels are low in primary and central hypothyroidism, normal in subclinical hypothyroidism, and high in peripheral thyroid hormone resistance

Additional Work-Up

Total triiodothyronine (T3) measurement	Less useful than T4 measurement because T3 level may be normal in patients with hypothyroidism
Measurement of thyroid peroxidase autoantibodies	These are often detectable in patients with Hashimoto thyroiditis (measurement is useful in patients with subclinical hypothyroidism)
Measurement of thyroglobulin autoantibodies	These are usually present with Hashimoto thyroiditis, although less so than thyroid peroxidase autoantibodies
Magnetic resonance imaging (MRI) of the brain and pituitary gland	If central hypothyroidism is present
Thyroid ultrasonography	If a thyroid nodule is detected on examination

Fine needle aspiration	To determine whether a palpable nodule is malignant
Measurement of luteinizing hormone (LH), follicle-stimulating hormone (FSH), cortisol level, prolactin, insulin-like growth factor I	If central hypothyroidism is diagnosed (to evaluate for hypopituitarism)
Thyrotropin-releasing hormone stimulating test	To distinguish secondary from tertiary hypothyroidism
Electrolyte measurements	Severe hypothyroidism may result in hyponatremia
Lipid panel	Hypothyroidism is associated with elevated triglycerides and elevated low-density lipoprotein cholesterol
Complete blood cell count	Hypothyroidism is associated with anemia
Fasting blood glucose measurement	To evaluate for diabetes

FURTHER READING

American Association of Clinical Endocrinologists: Medical guidelines for clinical practice for the evaluation and treatment of hyperthyroidism and hypothyroidism. Endocr Pract 2002;8:458-469.

Devdhar M, Ousman YH, Burman KD: Hypothyroidism. Endocrinol Metab Clin North Am 2007;36:595-615.

Hueston WJ: Treatment of hypothyroidism. Am Fam Physician 2001;64:1717-724.

Schmidt DN, Wallace K: How to diagnose hypopituitarism. Postgrad Med 1998;104(7):77-78, 81-87.

Wartofsky L, Van Nostrand D, Burman KD: Overt and "subclinical" hypothyroidism in women. Obstet Gynecol Surv 2006;61:535-542.

22 INFERTILITY

Theodore O'Connell

Infertility affects one couple in six and becomes more common as people age. Clinical evaluation of infertility is indicated if a pregnancy has not occurred after 1 year of regular unprotected intercourse. An infertility work-up should also be initiated in female patients who complain of infertility and have any of the following abnormalities: irregular menses or amenorrhea, bleeding between periods, dyspareunia, history of upper genital tract infection, history of a ruptured appendix or other abdominal surgery, or age older than 35 years.

Because men account for approximately 40% of all cases of infertility, the male partner should be evaluated early in the infertility work-up. Historical factors affecting the male partner should also be considered in determining when to begin an infertility evaluation. The following historical factors in the male partner warrant an early investigation: difficulty achieving or maintaining an erection; inability to ejaculate during intercourse; history of testicular injury, mumps, or an undescended testicle; or history of infection in the prostate gland, epididymis, or testicles.

There are several tests that every infertile couple should have performed. The first is a semen analysis of the male partner, regardless of how many pregnancies he has caused, because sperm counts can change over time. The second test is hysterosalpingography, which helps determine whether the uterine cavity is normal in size and shape and whether the fallopian tubes are patent. Although hysterosalpingography is the initial test to evaluate tubal patency, patients at high risk for infection, such as those with a history of clinically diagnosed pelvic inflammatory disease, are best evaluated initially with laparoscopy and hysteroscopy. Laparoscopy is more invasive than hysterosalpingography, but it remains the best test for identifying endometriosis and peritubal adhesions.

Routine hormonal assessment, especially in a young and apparently ovulatory patient, is controversial. There is less disagreement about performing a hormonal assessment in women aged 35 years and older. The suggested work-up is outlined later in this chapter.

In approximately 5% to 10% of infertile couples who proceed through a complete infertility evaluation, no cause is identified; these couples are said to have unexplained infertility. Infertility clinics may perform additional specialized testing, such as ultrasonography, testing for antisperm antibodies, and sperm function assays. Empirical treatment regimens have been designed to treat subtle disorders that may not be diagnosed.

Causes of Female Infertility

Endometriosis

Male factors

Ovulatory dysfunction
- Amenorrhea
- Hyperprolactinemia
- Oligomenorrhea

Tubal disease

Uterine causes
- Intrauterine synechiae (Asherman syndrome)
- Septate uterus
- Uterine fibroids

Unexplained infertilility

Key Historical Features

✓ Patient age

✓ Duration of infertility

✓ Timing of sexual intercourse

✓ Galactorrhea

✓ History of dyspareunia

✓ Age at menarche

✓ Intermenstrual bleeding

✓ Determination of whether the woman is currently having regular, monthly menstrual cycles

✓ Prior contraceptive use

✓ Reproductive history, especially previous pregnancies with the same male partner

✓ Medical history, especially thyroid disorders and diabetes mellitus

✓ Surgical history, especially appendectomy or other abdominal surgery

✓ Gynecologic history, especially sexually transmitted diseases, pelvic inflammatory disease, uterine fibroids, pelvic irradiation, or previous use of an intrauterine device

✓ Medications, especially oral contraceptives

✓ Family history, especially genetic diseases

✓ Cigarette smoking

✓   Caffeine use

✓   Alcohol use

✓   Illicit drug use

Key Physical Findings

✓   Height and weight

✓   Skin examination for acne or hirsutism

✓   Pelvic examination for evidence of infection, uterine fibroids, ovarian cysts, or endometriosis

✓   Genital examination of the male partner for phimosis, balanitis, testicular size, or evidence of testicular tumor

Suggested Work-Up

Semen analysis	To evaluate for a cause of infertility in the male partner
Hysterosalpingography	To evaluate the uterine cavity and determine whether the fallopian tubes are patent
Thyroid-stimulating hormone	To evaluate for thyroid disorders
Prolactin measurement	To evaluate for hyperprolactinemia
Measurement of estradiol and follicle-simulating hormone (FSH) level on cycle day 3	For patients aged 35 years and older to help determine ovarian reserve
	Elevated basal FSH levels higher than 8 to 10 mIU/mL are suggestive of declining fertility potential, and a concentration higher than 20 mIU/mL virtually excludes the chance of a spontaneous pregnancy
Measurement of serum progesterone on cycle day 21	A level above 10 ng/mL confirms that ovulation has occurred

Additional Work-Up

Basal body temperature measurement	May be used to help predict the timing of ovulation, but no longer

	recommended as part of the routine investigation of an infertile couple
Clomiphene citrate challenge test	May be used to increase the sensitivity of a basal FSH determination
	The FSH level is measured both before and after the administration of 100 mg of clomiphene citrate during days 5 through 9 of the menstrual cycle
	Elevation in the serum FSH level after the clomiphene citrate challenge indicates decreased ovarian reserve
Total testosterone and dehydroepiandrosterone sulfate levels	If signs of androgen excess are found on physical examination
Laparoscopy	Generally indicated in women with otherwise unexplained infertility and when there is evidence or suspicion of endometriosis, intrapelvic adhesions, or fallopian tube disease, particularly if the hysterosalpingogram is suggestive of tubal disease that may be amenable to surgical repair
Measurement of serum antibody to *Chlamydia trachomatis*	May be used as a screening tool for tubal pathologic conditions in infertile women
Routine cervical cultures	To identify active current chlamydia or gonorrhea infection in low-risk populations
Postcoital test	Indirectly measures cervical mucus competency
	Not routinely performed as part of the basic infertility evaluation because of marked variability in performance and variable interpretation

Endometrial biopsy	Provides an indirect measure of ovulation and evaluates the cumulative effect of progesterone on the endometrium; however, there is little role for routine endometrial biopsy as part of a general infertility evaluation
Sonohysterography	May be used as an alternative to hysterosalpingography to evaluate the uterine cavity but provides little information about the patency of the fallopian tubes
Magnetic resonance imaging	May be helpful in visualizing the uterine cavity and determining tubal patency

FURTHER READING

Brugh VM, Nudell DM, Lipshultz LI: What the urologist should know about the female infertility evaluation. Urol Clin North Am 2002;29:983-992.

Hargreave TB, Mills JA: Investigating and managing infertility in general practice. BMJ 1998;316:1438-1441.

Illions EH, Valley MT, Kaunitz AM: Infertility: a clinical guide for the internist. Med Clin North Am 1998;82:271-295.

Penzias AS: Infertility: contemporary office-based evaluation and treatment. Obstet Gynecol Clin 2000;27:473-486.

Smith S, Pfeifer SM, Collins JA: Diagnosis and management of female infertility. JAMA 2003;290:1767-1770.

Taylor A: ABC of subfertility: extent of the problem. BMJ 2003;327:434-436.

Kathleen Dor

The most common liver diseases during pregnancy are preeclampsia and viral hepatitis. Less common causes that are specific to pregnancy include intrahepatic cholestasis of pregnancy, acute fatty liver of pregnancy, Budd-Chiari syndrome, liver hematoma and rupture, and liver infarction.

In evaluating a patient with possible hepatic disease, liver cell damage is assessed by measurement of aspartate aminotransferase (AST) and alanine aminotransferase (ALT), whereas hepatic synthetic function is assessed by measurement of albumin level and prothrombin time (PT). Cholestatic disease is assessed by measurement of levels of alkaline phosphatase and bilirubin.

Acute fatty liver of pregnancy usually occurs late in pregnancy and is a medical emergency. It often manifests with nausea and vomiting, abdominal pain, headache, jaundice, and altered mental status. Acute fatty liver of pregnancy is associated with ALT levels lower than 500 IU/L; in acute viral hepatitis, in comparison, levels are often higher than 1000 IU/L. In addition, acute fatty liver of pregnancy is associated with disseminated intravascular coagulation, renal failure, pancreatitis, and hypoglycemia.

Intrahepatic cholestasis of pregnancy usually manifests initially with pruritus, followed by the development of jaundice. It is associated with elevations in serum bile acids (at least three times the normal level), bilirubin (<5 mg/dL), cholesterol and triglyceride levels, and normal or mildly elevated transaminase levels.

Budd-Chiari syndrome is the occlusion of the hepatic venous system and usually occurs in women with an underlying thrombophilia. This syndrome can occur at any time in pregnancy, and patients usually present with abdominal pain and distension, which progresses to ascites.

Medications Associated with Liver Disease

Angiotensin-converting enzyme (ACE) inhibitors

Acetaminophen

β blockers

Calcium channel blockers

Isoniazid

Ketoconazole

Methyldopa

Minocycline

Nitrofurantoin

Phenytoin

Pyrazinamide

Sulfonamides

Terbinafine

Causes of Liver Disease in Pregnancy

Acute fatty liver of pregnancy

Alcoholic hepatitis

Autoimmune hepatitis

Budd-Chiari syndrome

Cirrhosis

Eclampsia

Gallbladder disease

Syndrome of hemolysis, elevated liver enzyme counts, and low platelet count (HELLP)

Hyperemesis gravidarum

Intrahepatic cholestasis of pregnancy

Liver abscess

Liver adenoma

Liver hematoma and rupture

Liver infarction

Medications

Non-alcoholic fatty liver disease

Preeclampsia

Primary biliary cirrhosis

Primary sclerosing cholangitis

Viral hepatitis

Key Historical Features

✓   Headache

✓   Vision changes

✓   Facial and hand swelling (preeclampsia)

✓   Fever (cholangitis, acute viral hepatitis)

✓   Pruritus (intrahepatic cholestasis of pregnancy, primary biliary cirrhosis)

✓   Decreased appetite and fatigue (chronic liver disease)

- ✓ Gastrointestinal symptoms
  - Nausea and vomiting
  - Abdominal pain
  - Abdominal distension
  - Jaundice
  - Diarrhea
  - Rectal bleeding
  - Color of urine and stool
- ✓ Medical history, especially history of the following:
  - Liver disease
  - Previous episodes of jaundice
- ✓ Surgical history, especially previous biliary surgery
- ✓ Obstetric history
  - Most recent menstrual period
  - Previous ultrasonography during the pregnancy
  - Previous obstetric complications
- ✓ Medications
- ✓ Travel history
- ✓ Social history, including alcohol use, drug use, and sexual history

Key Physical Findings

- ✓ Vital signs
- ✓ Weight
- ✓ Examination for evidence of chronic liver disease: jaundice, scleral icterus, muscle mass loss, ascites, palmar erythema, spider angiomas, caput medusa, Dupuytren contracture, clubbing of digits
- ✓ Abdominal examination for hepatomegaly, splenomegaly, abdominal tenderness, or ascites
- ✓ Skin examination for excoriations that indicate pruritus
- ✓ Neurologic examination for evidence of hepatic encephalopathy

Suggested Work-Up

ALT, AST, bilirubin, and alkaline phosphatase measurements	To determine whether the liver disease is caused by hepatocyte damage or cholestasis

Serum bile acid measurements	To evaluate for intrahepatic cholestasis of pregnancy
Urinalysis	To evaluate for proteinuria
Complete blood cell count	To evaluate for anemia and thrombocytopenia, which are associated with liver disease
Blood urea nitrogen (BUN) and creatinine measurement	To evaluate for renal disease
Partial thromboplastin time (PTT), PT, and international normalized ratio (INR)	To evaluate for coagulopathy
Albumin measurement	To evaluate liver synthetic function
Serum electrolyte measurements	To evaluate for electrolyte abnormalities
Serum blood glucose measurement	To evaluate for hypo- or hyperglycemia

Additional Work-Up

Right upper quadrant ultrasonography	To evaluate the liver and gallbladder
Test for hepatitis A immunoglobulin M antibodies	To evaluate for acute hepatitis A infection
Test for hepatitis B surface antigen	To evaluate for hepatitis B infection (usually performed as a routine part of prenatal screening)
Test for hepatitis B core antibody	To evaluate for hepatitis B infection
Test for hepatitis C antibody	To evaluate for hepatitis C infection
Twenty-four-hour urine test for total protein	To evaluate for proteinuria (if preeclampsia is suspected)
Uric acid measurement	Elevated level is associated with preeclampsia

Lactate dehydrogenase measurement	Elevated level may be a sign of hemolysis associated with preeclampsia
Test for antimitochondrial antibody	To evaluate for primary biliary cirrhosis
Test for antinuclear antibody (ANA) and smooth muscle antibody	To evaluate for autoimmune hepatitis

FURTHER READING

Benjaminov FS, Heathcote J: Liver disease in pregnancy. Am J Gastroenterol 2004;99: 2479-2478.

Cappell MS. Hepatic and gastrointestinal diseases. In Gabbe SG, Niebyl JR, Simpson JL, eds: Obstetrics: Normal and Problem Pregnancies, 5th ed. New York: Churchill Livingstone, 2007, pp 1105-1115.

Hunt CM, Sharara AI: Liver disease in pregnancy. Am Fam Physician 1999;59:829-836.

Schutt VA, Minuk GY: Liver diseases unique to pregnancy. Best Pract Res Clin Gastroenterol 2007;21:771-792.

Teoh NC, Farrell GC: Liver disease caused by drugs. In Feldman M, Friedman LS, Brandt LJ, eds: Sleisenger & Fordtran's Gastrointestinal and Liver Disease, 8th ed. Philadelphia: Elsevier, 2006, pp 1807-1843.

NAUSEA AND VOMITING DURING PREGNANCY

Kathleen Dor

Nausea and vomiting of pregnancy, also known as *morning sickness*, is very common, affecting 70% to 85% of pregnant women. It can range in severity from mild nausea to hyperemesis gravidarum. The cause of nausea and vomiting of pregnancy is not known. Risk factors include molar gestation, multiple gestation, family history, or a history of hyperemesis gravidarum in prior pregnancies. Recognition and treatment of milder symptoms can prevent progression of symptoms and hospitalization.

Nausea and vomiting of pregnancy usually starts before 9 weeks of pregnancy and usually ends by the 20th week. If symptoms begin after 9 weeks, if the vomiting is severe, or if other symptoms are present, then other causes of nausea and vomiting should be investigated.

Medications That May Cause Nausea and Vomiting

Antibiotics

Cardiac antiarrhythmic agents

Chemotherapy agents

Digitalis

Estrogen

Levodopa

Morphine

Nicotine

Nonsteroidal anti-inflammatory drugs (NSAIDs)

Phenytoin

Progesterone

Causes of Nausea and Vomiting During Pregnancy*

Gastrointestinal disease

- Acute fatty liver of pregnancy
- Acute gastroenteritis
- Appendicitis

*Adapted from Goodwin TM. Hyperemesis Gravidarum. *Clinical Obstetrics and Gynecology* 1998; 41: 597-605, Table 1.

- Biliary tract disease
- Bowel obstruction
- Gastric cancer
- Gastroesophageal reflux disease
- Hepatitis
- Pancreatitis
- Peptic ulcer disease

Genitourinary disease

- Nephrolithiasis
- Ovarian torsion
- Pyelonephritis

Hyperemesis gravidarum

Nausea and vomiting of pregnancy (first trimester)

Preeclampsia

Medications

Metabolic disease

- Addison disease
- Diabetic ketoacidosis
- Hyperthyroidism
- Uremia

Neurologic disease

- Benign positional vertigo
- Brain tumor
- Encephalitis
- Intracranial hemorrhage
- Meningitis
- Migraine headache

Key Historical Features

✓ Gravity and parity

✓ Onset of symptoms

✓ Frequency and severity

✓ History of nausea and vomiting with other pregnancies

✓ Presence of diarrhea

✓ Abdominal pain

✓ Significant weight loss associated with vomiting

✓ Fever and chills, which may indicate infection such as cholecystitis, pyelonephritis, or appendicitis

✓ Palpitations, heat intolerance, or anxiety, which may indicate hyperthyroidism

✓ Medical history, especially history of thyroid disease, liver disease, gallbladder disease, pancreatitis, gastroesophageal reflux disease, migraines, or diabetes

✓ Medications

✓ Family history

- A family history of diabetes mellitus, thyroid disease, or migraines, which can increase the risk for these diseases

- Similar symptoms in other family members, in which case an infectious cause should be considered, such as acute gastroenteritis

✓ Social history

- Alcohol abuse, which can cause pancreatitis

- Drug use

- Tobacco use

✓ Review of systems, especially the following:

- Gastrointestinal symptoms

    — Vomiting that begins after the 9th week of pregnancy, which is usually not part of clinical nausea and vomiting of pregnancy

    — Diarrhea, which may indicate gastroenteritis or hyperthyroidism

    — Abdominal pain, which may indicate an intra-abdominal process such as cholecystitis, pancreatitis, appendicitis, or bowel obstruction

- Genitourinary symptoms

    — Dysuria, which may indicate a urinary tract infection

    — Hematuria, which may indicate nephrolithiasis or a urinary tract infection

- Neurologic symptoms

    — Headaches, which may be suggestive of a migraine, meningitis, or brain tumor

Key Physical Findings

✓ Vital signs

- Fever

- Hypotension, which can be indicative of severe dehydration or sepsis
- Hypertension, which can be indicative of preeclampsia

✓ General assessment of health and well-being

✓ Neurologic examination to evaluate for a central nervous system disorder

✓ Head and neck examination

- Facial edema may be suggestive of preeclampsia
- Dry mucous membranes, which indicate dehydration
- Photophobia, which may indicate a central nervous system process
- Neck stiffness, which may indicate meningitis
- A goiter, which indicates thyroid disease

✓ Cardiovascular examination for tachycardia, which may indicate dehydration, infection, or hyperthyroidism

✓ Gastrointestinal examination

- Abdominal tenderness, which may indicate an intra-abdominal process, such as cholecystitis, pancreatitis, appendicitis, or bowel obstruction
- An enlarged liver, which indicates liver disease

✓ Back examination for costovertebral angle tenderness, which is suggestive of pyelonephritis

✓ Extremity examination for edema, suggestive of preeclampsia

✓ Skin examination

- Jaundice, suggestive of liver or biliary tract disease
- Poor skin turgor, suggestive of dehydration

Suggested Work-Up

Pregnancy test	To confirm pregnancy if not already done
Urinalysis	For ketonuria and a high specific gravity, which indicate dehydration
	For pyuria, which indicates possible urinary tract infection
	For glucosuria, which indicates hyperglycemia and possible diabetes
	For proteinuria, which may indicate preeclampsia

Additional Work-Up

Further workup should be guided by the patient's symptoms and the physical examination. If the timing, persistence, and severity of symptoms are not suggestive of typical nausea and vomiting of pregnancy, a further work up is necessary:

Serum glucose measurement	If diabetes mellitus is suspected
Complete blood cell count	To evaluate for infection such as cholecystitis or pyelonephritis
Blood urea nitrogen (BUN) and creatinine measurement	To evaluate for dehydration or renal disease
Serum electrolyte measurements	For hypokalemia or hyponatremia in cases of severe vomiting
	To evaluate for the development of acidosis in patients with severe dehydration
Liver enzyme measurements	If hepatitis is suspected
Bilirubin measurement	If gallbladder or liver disease is suspected
Amylase or lipase measurement	If pancreatitis is suspected
Thyroid-stimulating hormone (TSH)	If thyroid disease is suspected
Abdominal ultrasonography	If liver, gallbladder, or pancreatic disease is suspected
Obstetric ultrasonography	If multiple fetuses or molar disease is suspected
Esophagogastroduodenoscopy	If peptic ulcer disease is suspected

FURTHER READING

American College of Obstetrics and Gynecology: ACOG (American College of Obstetrics and Gynecology) Practice Bulletin: nausea and vomiting of pregnancy. Obstet Gynecol 2004;103:803-814.

Goodwin TM: Hyperemesis gravidarum. Clin Obstet Gynecol 1998;41:597-605.

Koch KL, Frissora CL: Nausea and vomiting during pregnancy. Gastroenterol Clin 2003;32:201-234.

Kuşcu NK, Koyuncu F: Hyperemesis gravidarum: current concepts and management. Postgrad Med J 2002;78(916):76-79.

Quinlan JD, Hill DA: Nausea and vomiting of pregnancy. Am Fam Physician 2003;68: 121-128.

25 OSTEOPOROSIS

Theodore O'Connell

Primary osteoporosis results from deterioration of bone mass that is related to aging and decreased gonadal function but is not associated with any chronic illness. Because primary osteoporosis results from decreased gonadal function, early menopause or premenopausal estrogen deficiency may hasten the development of osteoporosis in women. Other risk factors for primary osteoporosis include female gender in general, white or Asian ancestry, sedentary lifestyle, tobacco use, low calcium intake, and low body weight.

Secondary osteoporosis results from chronic conditions that contribute to accelerated loss of bone density. Chronic conditions that may contribute to secondary osteoporosis include acromegaly, alcoholism, anorexia nervosa, chronic liver disease, diabetes mellitus type I, glycogen storage diseases, hemochromatosis, homocystinuria, hyperadrenocorticism, hyperparathyroidism, hyperprolactinemia, hypophosphatasia, malabsorption syndromes and gastric bypass surgery, Marfan syndrome, osteogenesis imperfecta, renal disease, thyrotoxicosis, and vitamin D deficiency.

Men are more likely than women to have a secondary cause of osteoporosis. In the patient with osteoporosis, initial evaluation should begin with a risk factor assessment (see risk factors listed later in this chapter), documentation of history, and a physical examination focusing on signs of chronic disease. If secondary osteoporosis is suspected on the basis of findings from the history and physical examination, a work-up should be performed.

Long-term glucocorticoid therapy is a common cause of osteoporosis. Medications that may cause osteoporosis are listed below.

Medications Associated with Osteoporosis

Cyclosporine

Glucocorticoids

Gonadotropin-releasing hormone (GnRH) agonists

Heparin (prolonged treatment)

Methotrexate

Phenobarbital

Phenothiazines

Phenytoin

Thyroid hormone excess

Risk Factors for Osteoporosis

Advancing age

Alcohol abuse

White or Asian race

Chronic kidney disease

Early menopause

Family history of osteoporosis

Female gender

High caffeine intake

Impaired calcium absorption

Late menarche

Low intake of calcium, phosphorus, or vitamin D

Nulliparity

Low body weight or small body frame

Sedentary lifestyle

Tobacco use

Suggested Work-Up for Patients with Suspected Secondary Osteoporosis

Serum creatinine measurement	To evaluate for renal disease
Alanine transaminase (ALT) and aspartate transaminase (AST) measurement	To evaluate for liver disease
Alkaline phosphatase measurement	To evaluate for liver disease, Paget disease, or other bone pathologic processes
Albumin measurement	To evalvate for malnutrition
Serum calcium measurement	Decreased level may indicate malabsorption or vitamin D deficiency; increased level may indicate primary hyperparathyroidism or malignancy
Serum iron and ferritin measurements	Levels are increased with hemochromatosis

Serum phosphorus measurement	Decreased level may indicate osteomalacia
Thyroid-stimulating hormone (TSH) measurement	To evaluate for hyperthyroidism
Serum protein electrophoresis (SPEP), measurement of erythrocyte sedimentation rate (ESR), complete blood cell count (CBC), serum calcium measurement, parathyroid hormone (PTH) measurement	Abnormal SPEP, elevated ESR, anemia, hypercalcemia, and depressed parathyroid hormone level are suggestive of multiple myeloma
Estrogen level measurement	Decreased levels in premenopausal women are suggestive of hypogonadism
1,25-Hydroxyvitamin D measurement	Elevated levels occur with hyperparathyroidism
25-Hydroxycalciferol measurement	Decreased levels suggest vitamin D deficiency
24-hour urine calcium measurement	Decreased urinary calcium excretion is suggestive of malabsorption or vitamin D deficiency

Additional Work-Up

Dexamethasone suppression test	May be indicated when Cushing syndrome is suspected
Stool fat quantification or xylose breath test	Used when there is a history of gastrectomy or diarrhea to evaluate for malabsorption

FURTHER READING

Harper KD, Weber TJ: Secondary osteoporosis. Diagnostic considerations. Endocrinol Metab Clin North Am 1998;27:325-348.

Kenny AM, Prestwood KM: Osteoporosis: pathogenesis, diagnosis, and treatment in older adults. Rheum Dis Clin North Am 2000;26:569-591.

Simon LS: Osteoporosis. Clin Geriatr Med 2005;21:603-629, viii.

South-Paul, JE: Osteoporosis: part I: evaluation and assessment. Am Fam Physician 2001;63:897-904.

Tresolini CP, Gold DT, Lee LS, eds: Working with Patients to Prevent, Treat and Manage Osteoporosis: A Curriculum Guide for Health Professions, 2nd ed. San Francisco: National Fund for Medical Education, 1998.

Kathleen Dor

Acute pelvic pain is pain felt in the pelvic area for less than 48 hours. It can be difficult to make the diagnosis on the basis of history and physical examination alone, because acute pelvic pain can have gynecologic, obstetric, urologic, musculoskeletal, or gastrointestinal causes. When a patient with acute pelvic pain initially presents for evaluation, it is important to quickly determine whether the patient is pregnant and whether the patient has a surgical emergency.

Pelvic inflammatory disease should be considered as a cause in all patients who are sexually active. Aggressive diagnosis and appropriate treatment in adolescent patients are important in order to avoid the long-term sequelae of pelvic inflammatory disease, including infertility, chronic pelvic pain, and ectopic pregnancy. Ectopic pregnancy also should be considered in all sexually active patients with acute pelvic or abdominal pain.

Causes of Acute Pelvic Pain

Gastrointestinal

Appendicitis

Bowel obstruction

Colitis

Diverticulitis

Gastroenteritis

Hernia

Irritable bowel syndrome

Mesenteric lymphadenitis

Volvulus

Gynecologic

Dysmenorrhea

Endometriosis

Gynecologic neoplasm

Hemorrhagic ovarian cyst

Misplaced intrauterine device (IUD)

Mittelschmerz

Ovarian cyst rupture

Ovarian cyst torsion

Pelvic abscess

Pelvic inflammatory disease

Sexual assault/trauma

Uterine fibroids

Uterine perforation

Musculoskeletal

Hip fracture

Muscle strain

Pelvic fracture

Psoas abscess

Spinal neoplasm

Obstetric

Ectopic pregnancy

Labor

Placental abruption

Preterm labor

Round ligament pain

Spontaneous abortion

Septic abortion

Urinary

Urinary tract infection

Urinary tract stone

Other

Diabetic ketoacidosis

Pelvic thrombophlebitis

Shingles

Key Historical Features

✓   General

- Fevers and chills, which may indicate infection
- Decreased appetite, which may indicate peritonitis
- Quality, onset, location, and duration of pain

- Increased thirst and weight loss, which may indicate diabetes
- History of recent trauma or assault

✓ Gynecologic

- Prior episodes of similar pain and association with menses
- Most recent normal menstrual period
- Vaginal discharge, which may indicate pelvic inflammatory disease
- Sexual history
- Prior surgery
- Prior sexually transmitted diseases (STDs)
- Previous pregnancies, including ectopic pregnancies
- Recent miscarriages or therapeutic abortions
- Contraceptive method, especially IUD

✓ Gastrointestinal

- Nausea and vomiting, which may indicate obstruction, appendicitis, gastroenteritis, or urinary tract stone
- Prior abdominal surgery, which increases the risk for bowel obstruction
- History of diverticulitis or findings of diverticular disease on prior colonoscopy
- Absence of bowel movements, which may indicate bowel obstruction

✓ Urologic

- Dysuria, hematuria, or urinary frequency or urgency, which may indicate a urinary tract infection; dysuria may also indicate a sexually transmitted disease

Key Physical Findings

✓ Vital signs, especially for signs of dehydration, sepsis, infection, or severe blood loss

✓ General appearance

✓ Gastrointestinal examination

- Inspection of the abdomen for distension, scars, or hernias
- Palpation of the abdomen for tenderness, guarding, or rebound, which may indicate peritonitis
- Palpation of the abdomen for masses
- Auscultation of the abdomen for bowel sounds, the absence of which may indicate peritonitis or obstruction

- • Rectal examination to evaluate for rectal bleeding, masses, or tenderness
- ✓ Gynecologic examination
    - • Examination of the external genitalia for lesions or tenderness
    - • Single-finger vaginal examination for areas of tenderness
    - • Bimanual examination to examine the uterus and adnexa for tenderness, masses, or evidence of pregnancy
    - • Speculum examination to inspect the vaginal mucosa and cervix, especially for blood, discharge, or lesions and to determine whether the cervical os is open or closed
- ✓ Musculoskeletal examination
    - • Palpation of the back to evaluate for areas of tenderness
    - • Evaluation of the back for range of motion and any obvious masses or deformities
- ✓ Skin examination to evaluate for any skin lesions that may indicate shingles

Suggested Work-Up

Urine pregnancy test	To evaluate for pregnancy
Cervical culture/swab for *Neisseria gonorrhoeae* and *Chlamydia trachomatis*	To evaluate for gonorrhea and chlamydia infection
Complete blood cell count	To evaluate for infection or anemia
Chemistry panel	To evaluate for dehydration or acidosis
Urinalysis	To evaluate for urinary tract infection, urinary tract stones, or diabetic ketoacidosis

Additional Work-Up

Urine culture	If a urinary tract infection is suspected
Pelvic ultrasonography	If the patient is pregnant or gynecologic disease is suspected
Quantitative β–human chorionic gonadotropin measurement	If the urine pregnancy test yields positive results and an intrauterine

	pregnancy is not seen on ultrasonography
Blood culture	If sepsis is suspected
Computed tomographic (CT) scan of abdomen and pelvis	If the examination findings suggest appendicitis, diverticulitis, urinary tract stone, or abscess (pregnancy test should be performed before CT scanning is done)
Abdominal radiography	If bowel obstruction or urinary tract stone is suspected (pregnancy test should be performed first)
Blood typing and screening	If the patient is pregnant to evaluate whether patient is Rh negative

FURTHER READING

Baines PA, Allen GM: Pelvic pain and menstrual related illness. Emerg Med Clin North Am 2001;19:763-780.

Hewitt GD, Brown RT: Acute and chronic pelvic pain in female adolescents. Med Clin North Am 2000;84:1009-1025.

Samraj GPN, Curry RW Jr: Acute pelvic pain: evaluation and management. Compr Ther 2004;30:173-184.

Kathleen Dor

Chronic pelvic pain is defined as noncyclic pelvic pain that has lasted 6 or more months. The additional requirement of severity enough to cause functional disability or to necessitate medical or surgical treatment is often used in the definition. *Pelvic pain* may refer to pain that localizes to the pelvis, lower abdominal wall, lower back, or buttocks. About 15% to 20% of 18- to 50-year-old women suffer from chronic pelvic pain.

The most common causes of chronic pelvic pain are endometriosis, interstitial cystitis, adhesions, and irritable bowel syndrome. In addition, there is a strong association between chronic pelvic pain and a history of physical or sexual abuse.

The cause of chronic pelvic pain is often not discernible even after thorough evaluation. In addition, there may be several associated conditions that contribute to the pelvic pain. Disorders of the reproductive tract, gastrointestinal system, urologic organs, musculoskeletal system, and neurologic system, as well as psychologic factors, may be associated with chronic pelvic pain in women. On occasion, only one of these disorders is present, and treatment is curative. More often, however, the pain is associated with several diagnoses, and a number of contributing factors necessitate evaluation and treatment.

Causes of Chronic Pelvic Pain

Gastrointestinal

Celiac disease

Chronic intermittent bowel obstruction

Colitis

Colon cancer

Constipation

Diverticular disease

Hernias

Inflammatory bowel disease

Irritable bowel syndrome

Gynecologic

Adenomyosis

Adhesions

Cervical stenosis

151

Chronic ectopic pregnancy

Chronic endometritis

Chronic pelvic inflammatory disease

Endometrial or cervical polyps

Endometriosis

Endosalpingiosis

Intrauterine contraceptive device

Malignancies

Ovarian cysts

Ovarian remnant syndrome

Ovarian retention syndrome

Ovulatory pain

Pelvic congestion syndrome

Postoperative peritoneal cysts

Symptomatic pelvic relaxation

Tuberculous salpingitis

Uterine fibroids

Musculoskeletal

Abdominal wall pain

Chronic coccygeal pain

Compression fracture

Degenerative joint disease

Disk herniation

Fibromyalgia

Low back pain

Muscle strain or sprain

Neuralgia of iliohypogastric, ilioinguinal, or genitofemoral nerves

Pelvic floor myalgia

Piriformis syndrome

Poor posture

Rectus tendon strain

Spinal cord or sacral nerve cancer

Spondylosis

Urologic

Bladder cancer

Chronic urinary tract infection

Cystitis (interstitial or radiation)

Recurrent acute cystitis

Recurrent acute urethritis

Uninhibited bladder contractions

Urethral caruncle

Urethral diverticulum

Urethral syndrome

Urinary tract stone

Miscellaneous

Abdominal cutaneous nerve entrapment in surgical scar

Abdominal epilepsy

Abdominal migraine

Bipolar personality disorder

Depression

Familial Mediterranean fever

Neurologic dysfunction

Shingles

Sleep disturbances

Somatic referral

Key Historical Features

✓ Location, timing, and quality of pain

✓ Associated fever, chills, or night sweats, which may indicate infection or cancer

✓ Associated weight loss, which may indicate cancer

✓ Associated increased abdominal girth, which may indicate a mass or ascites

✓ History of physical or sexual abuse

✓ Medical history

- Especially interstitial cystitis, irritable bowel syndrome, pelvic inflammatory disease, or endometriosis

✓ Surgical history

✓ Obstetric and gynecologic history

- Previous pregnancies

- History of infertility, which may indicate endometriosis or chronic pelvic inflammatory disease

- Menstrual symptoms and associated pain
- Pain associated with intercourse
- History of sexually transmitted diseases or pelvic inflammatory disease
- Birth control method

✓ Prior gynecologic surgeries

✓ Social history
- Alcohol or drug abuse
- Tobacco use

✓ Review of systems, especially the following:
- Gastrointestinal symptoms
  — Symptoms suggestive of irritable bowel syndrome such as constipation or diarrhea or both, abdominal distension, relief of pain with bowel movements, or mucus in bowel movements
  — Rectal bleeding
- Urologic symptoms
  — Dysuria, urinary urgency, or frequency, which may indicate interstitial cystitis or infection
  — Hematuria, which may indicate bladder neoplasm or infection
  — A history of recurrent urinary tract infections associated with negative culture results, which may indicate interstitial cystitis

✓ Psychologic
- History of depression or symptoms of depression

Key Physical Findings

✓ Vital signs
✓ General assessment of health for evidence of weight loss
✓ Abdominal examination
- Inspection of the abdomen for scars
- Palpation of the abdomen for organomegaly, masses, or tenderness
- Rectal examination
- Evaluation for hernias

✓ Gynecologic examination
- Examination of the external genitalia for lesions or tenderness
- Single-finger vaginal examination for areas of tenderness
- Bimanual examination to evaluate the uterus and adnexa
- Speculum examination to inspect the vaginal mucosa and cervix

✓ Musculoskeletal examination
  • Palpation of the back to evaluate for areas of tenderness
  • Evaluation of the back for range of motion and any obvious masses or deformities
✓ Skin examination for any skin lesions that may indicate shingles

Suggested Work-Up

The work-up of patients with chronic pelvic pain should be guided by the history and physical examination:

Urine pregnancy test or serum β—human chorionic gonadotropin	To rule out pregnancy
Transvaginal pelvic ultrasonography	To evaluate for pelvic masses
Pap smear	To evaluate for cervical dysplasia
Swab/culture for *Neisseria gonorrhoeae* and *Chlamydia* organisms	To evaluate for pelvic inflammatory disease
Urinalysis and urine culture	To evaluate for microscopic hematuria and urinary infections
Complete blood cell count	To evaluate for infection

Additional Work-Up

Depending on the history and physical examination, as well as findings from the initial evaluation, a more extensive workup may be warranted:

Computed tomographic (CT) scan of abdomen and pelvis	To further evaluate abnormal findings on pelvic ultrasonography or examination
Laparoscopy	To evaluate for endometriosis, adhesions, or pelvic masses or neoplasms
Cystoscopy	To evaluate for interstitial cystitis if symptoms are suggestive of this diagnosis and to evaluate for bladder neoplasms if microscopic hematuria is present

Intravesical potassium sensitivity test	If interstitial cystitis is suspected
Flexible sigmoidoscopy or colonoscopy	To evaluate for colonic neoplasms
Magnetic resonance imaging (MRI) of spine	If disease of the spine is suspected

FURTHER READING

ACOG Committee on Practice Bulletins–Gynecology: ACOG Practice Bulletin No. 51. Chronic pelvic pain. Obstet Gynecol 2004;103:589-605.

Bordman R, Jackson B: Below the belt: approach to chronic pelvic pain. Can Fam Physician 2006;52:1556-1562.

Gunter J: Chronic pelvic pain: an integrated approach to diagnosis and treatment. Obstet Gynecol Surv 2003;58:615-623.

Howard FM: Chronic pelvic pain. Obstet Gynecol 2003;101:594-611.

POLYCYSTIC OVARY SYNDROME

Kathleen Dor

Polycystic ovary syndrome (PCOS) is the most common endocrine disorder in women of reproductive age. Women with PCOS often have irregular menses, obesity, infertility, and hirsutism.

Diagnostic criteria from the 2003 meeting of the European Society of Human Reproduction and Embryology/American Society for Reproductive Medicine (ESHRE/ASRM) stressed that PCOS could be diagnosed only if other causes of hyperandrogenism were ruled out; such causes include androgen-secreting tumors, Cushing syndrome, and congenital adrenal hyperplasia. In addition, two of three criteria must be present to make the diagnosis: oligo-ovulation or anovulation, signs of hyperandrogenism, and ultrasound evidence of polycystic ovaries. These newer criteria include atypical manifestations of PCOS.

PCOS is a worrisome disease because of the potential complications. Women with PCOS are at higher risk for infertility, first-trimester miscarriages, endometrial hyperplasia (with chronic anovulation), type 2 diabetes mellitus, dyslipidemia, and cardiovascular disease. These complications can be treated and prevented; therefore, it is important to diagnose PCOS.

Medications That May Cause Symptoms That Mimic Polycystic Ovary Syndrome

Anabolic steroids (may cause hirsutism, acne, and amenorrhea)

Danazol (may cause amenorrhea and hirsutism)

Diazoxide (may cause hirsutism)

Glucocorticoids (may cause hirsutism)

Oral contraceptives (may cause amenorrhea)

Phenytoin (may cause hirsutism)

Progestins (may cause amenorrhea, hirsutism, and acne)

Testosterone (may cause amenorrhea, hirsutism, and acne)

Causes of Polycystic Ovary Syndrome

The cause of polycystic ovary syndrome is not completely understood. It involves the dysregulation of complex hormone cycles that leads to luteinizing hormone excess, androgen excess, insulin resistance, and chronic anovulation. There is a probable genetic predisposition to PCOS that is affected by environmental factors, especially obesity.

Key Historical Features:

✓ Medical history

- Type 2 diabetes mellitus, hyperlipidemia, hypertension, hyperprolactinemia, or thyroid disease

✓ Medications

✓ Menstrual history

- Irregular menses or amenorrhea (may be present in patients with PCOS)
- Secondary amenorrhea (may also indicate pregnancy or hyperprolactinemia)

✓ Reproductive history

- Anovulatory cycles in PCOS (results in infertility)
- When pregnancy does occur, higher risk for recurrent first-trimester miscarriages

✓ Family history

- PCOS, type diabetes mellitus, hypertension, hyperlipidemia, thyroid disease, and nonclassical congenital adrenal hyperplasia

✓ Constitutional symptoms

- Fatigue, cold intolerance, and constipation (may indicate hypothyroidism)
- Palpitations, heat intolerance, anxiety, diarrhea, and weight loss (may indicate hyperthyroidism)

✓ Skin symptoms

- Hirsutism and acne (indicative of hyperandrogenism)
- Dry skin and brittle hair (may be suggestive of hypothyroidism)

✓ Neurologic symptoms

- Headaches and visual disturbance (may be suggestive of a pituitary tumor)

Key Physical Findings

✓ Vital signs

✓ General assessment

- Obesity (in PCOS is central in distribution)
- Moon facies or a buffalo hump (can be suggestive of Cushing syndrome)

- Deepening of the voice (a sign of virilization and is a red flag for an androgen-secreting tumor)
- Acromegaly (suggestive of a pituitary tumor)

✓ Head and neck examination

- Visual field defect (suggestive of a pituitary tumor)
- Goiter (suggestive of hypothyroidism)

✓ Cardiovascular

- Hypertension (can be indicative of underlying cardiovascular disease, metabolic syndrome, or Cushing syndrome)
- Bradycardia (may be suggestive of hypothyroidism)
- Tachycardia (may be suggestive of hyperthyroidism)

✓ Skin examination

- Acanthosis nigricans (associated with insulin resistance)
- Abdominal striae and easy bruising (can be indicative of Cushing syndrome)
- Hirsutism and acne (indicative of hyperandrogenism)
- Male-pattern alopecia (rare in PCOS and could be suggestive of an androgen-secreting neoplasm)

✓ Pelvic and vaginal examination

- Palpable enlargement of ovaries, as a result of ovarian cysts
- Clitoromegaly (a sign of virilization)

Suggested Work-Up

The key to evaluating for PCOS is to rule out other diseases that can cause similar signs and symptoms:

Pregnancy test	To rule out pregnancy
Serum prolactin level measurement	To evaluate for hyperprolactinemia/pituitary adenoma
Fasting blood glucose measurement or glucose tolerance test	To evaluate for diabetes or glucose intolerance
Fasting lipid panel	To evaluate for hyperlipidemia
Thyroid-stimulating hormone measurement	To evaluate for hyper- or hypothyroidism
Dehydroepiandrosterone sulfate (DHEAS)	To evaluate for hyperandrogenism and rule out an androgen-producing tumor

| Free testosterone | To evaluate for hyperandrogenism and rule out an androgen-producing tumor |

Additional Work-Up

On the basis of the history and physical examination and the results of the tests just listed, a more extensive work-up may be warranted:

Pelvic ultrasonography	To evaluate for cystic ovaries, ideally performed on cycle days 3, 4, or 5 and with a vaginal probe
Total testosterone measurement	To evaluate for hyperandrogenism and rule out an androgen-producing tumor
Androstenedione measurement	To evaluate for hyperandrogenism
Serum 17-hydroxyprogesterone measurement	To evaluate for non-classic congenital adrenal hyperplasia
Dexamethasone suppression test	If Cushing syndrome is suspected
Twenty-four-hour urine cortisol measurement	If Cushing syndrome is suspected
Luteinizing hormone (LH) and follicle-stimulating hormone (FSH) measurements	For a high LH/FSH ratio, which is suggestive of PCOS (usually 3:1 or higher)
Estradiol level measurement	A low estradiol level in conjunction with a high FSH level is suggestive of premature ovarian failure in a patient with amenorrhea
Fasting insulin measurement	To evaluate for insulin resistance (a ratio of fasting glucose to insulin of 4.5 or lower indicates insulin resistance)
Endometrial biopsy	If endometrial hyperplasia or carcinoma is suspected

FURTHER READING

Buccola JM, Reynolds EE: Polycystic ovary syndrome: a review for primary providers. Prim Care Clin Office Pract 2003;30:697-710.

Buggs C, Rosenfield RL: Polycystic ovary syndrome in adolescence. Endocrinol Metab Clin 2005;34:677-705.

Carmina E: The spectrum of androgen excess disorders. Fertil Steril 2006;85:1582-1585.

Habif TP: Clinical Dermatology, 4th ed, St. Louis: Mosby, 2004.

Hart R, Norman R: Polycystic ovarian syndrome—prognosis and outcomes. Best Pract Res Clin Obstet Gynaecol 2006;20:751-778.

Richardson MR: Current perspectives in polycystic ovary syndrome. Am Fam Physician 2003;68:697-704.

The Rotterdam ESHRE/ASRM–Sponsored PCOS Consensus Workshop Group: Revised 2003 consensus on diagnostic criteria and long-term health risks related to polycystic ovary syndrome (PCOS). Hum Reprod 2004;19(1):41-47.

29 POSTMENOPAUSAL VAGINAL BLEEDING

Theodore O'Connell

Postmenopausal bleeding may be defined as vaginal bleeding starting 12 months or more after the cessation of menses or unscheduled bleeding in a postmenopausal woman who has been taking hormone replacement therapy for 12 months or more. All women with postmenopausal bleeding should be evaluated for potential malignancy, including endometrial cancer, premalignant atypical endometrial hyperplasia, and cervical cancer.

No universal algorithm exists for proceeding with an evaluation of a woman with postmenopausal bleeding. Tissue sampling is the most definitive diagnostic procedure. However, because up to 90% of postmenopausal bleeding has a benign cause, questions have arisen regarding the appropriateness of biopsy in all patients with postmenopausal bleeding. Imaging techniques, particularly transvaginal ultrasonography, have been explored to help determine which patients are at higher risk of malignancy and would benefit from tissue sampling and which patients are more likely to have a benign cause for the bleeding.

The use of transvaginal ultrasonography has been studied most extensively in postmenopausal women. In the absence of visible anomalies such as fibroids, endometrial thickness has been used as a marker for endometrial disease. In postmenopausal women, 5 mm of endometrial thickness is the most commonly used threshold; this marker has been shown to be 96% sensitive for endometrial carcinoma and 92% for other endometrial disease. The sensitivities are not significantly different in women taking hormone replacement therapy. An abnormal ultrasound result must be followed by either tissue sampling or saline-infusion sonography.

Many studies have shown that a threshold of 5 mm for pursuing endometrial sampling reasonably excludes patients with endometrial carcinoma. Some authors have suggested a thicker threshold for ruling out endometrial adenocarcinoma. However, cases of endometrial carcinoma have been detected in women with an endometrial thickness of as little as 3 mm. Therefore, a threshold of 5 mm is most commonly used.

Other techniques have been proposed to add accuracy to the imaging of the endometrium. Saline-infusion sonohysterography has been used in the evaluation of postmenopausal bleeding because the infusion of saline into the endometrial cavity may improve the differentiation of intraluminal masses and shape of the endometrium.

Hysteroscopy is the "gold standard" for the evaluation of postmenopausal bleeding because of the ability to perform directed biopsy. The limitations of hysteroscopy are the invasive nature of the procedure, the requirement for expensive equipment, and the risks associated with general anesthesia.

Three-dimensional ultrasonography is a technique with emerging applications that has been used for evaluation of postmenopausal bleeding. The actual benefit of three-dimensional imaging in most patients is probably limited.

Medications Linked to Postmenopausal Vaginal Bleeding

Anticoagulants

Antipsychotics

Corticosteroids

Herbal and other supplements

Hormonal contraception

Hormone replacement

Intrauterine devices

Selective serotonin reuptake inhibitors

Tamoxifen

Thyroid hormone replacement

Causes of Postmenopausal Vaginal Bleeding

Adenomyosis

Adrenal hyperplasia and Cushing disease

Atrophic endometrium

Bleeding disorders, including von Willebrand disease

Cervical carcinoma

Cervical dysplasia

Cervical polyp

Cervicitis

Endometrial carcinoma

Endometrial hyperplasia

Endometrial polyp

Endometritis

Estrogen-producing ovarian tumors

Leiomyomata

Leiomyosarcoma

Leukemia

Liver failure

Medications and herbal supplements

Myometritis

Renal disease

Salpingitis

Testosterone-producing ovarian tumors

Thrombocytopenia

Trauma (foreign body, abrasions, lacerations, sexual abuse or assault)

Key Historical Features

✓ Frequency, duration, and severity of flow

✓ Postcoital bleeding

✓ Pelvic pain

✓ Easy bruising or tendency to bleed

✓ Jaundice or history of hepatitis

✓ Medical history

✓ Surgical history

✓ Obstetric and gynecologic history

✓ Medications

Key Physical Findings

✓ Vital signs

✓ Pelvic examination to evaluate for vulvar or vaginal lesions, signs of trauma, cervical polyps or dysplasia, uterine enlargement, or adnexal masses

Suggested Work-Up

Pap smear is necessary to evaluate for cervical disease. Endometrial evaluation may include one or more of the following:

Transvaginal ultrasonography (with biopsy if the endometrial thickness is greater than 5 mm)

Saline-infusion sonohysterography with endometrial biopsy

Hysteroscopy with biopsy

Dilatation and curettage

No universal algorithm exists for proceeding with an evaluation of a woman with postmenopausal bleeding. Tissue sampling is the most definitive diagnostic procedure, but the techniques have variable sensitivity and specificity. Further research is necessary to determine the best method for evaluating the endometrium in patients with abnormal uterine bleeding.

Additional Work-Up

Cultures for *Neisseria gonorrhoeae* and *Chlamydia* organisms	If infection is suspected or if the patient is at risk for sexually transmitted disease
Complete blood cell count (CBC)	If anemia is suspected
Liver function tests and prothrombin time measurement	If liver disease is suspected
CBC with platelet count, prothrombin time measurement, and partial thromboplastin time measurement	If coagulopathy is suspected
von Willebrand factor assay	If von Willebrand disease is suspected

FURTHER READING

Albers JR, Hull SH, Wesley RM: Abnormal uterine bleeding. Am Fam Physician 2004;69:1915-1926.

Chen BH, Giudice LC: Dysfunctional uterine bleeding. West J Med 1998;169:280-284.

Davidson KG, Dubinsky TJ: Ultrasonographic evaluation of the endometrium in postmenopausal vaginal bleeding. Radiol Clin North Am 2003;41:769-780.

Goldstein SR: Abnormal uterine bleeding: the role of ultrasound. Radiol Clin North Am 2005;44:901-910.

Kilbourn C, Richards C: Abnormal uterine bleeding. Postgrad Med 2001;109(1):137-140.

Lethaby A, Farquhar C, Sarkis A, et al: Hormone replacement therapy in postmenopausal women: endometrial hyperplasia and irregular bleeding. Cochrane Database Syst Rev 2003;(4):CD000402.

Schrager S: Abnormal uterine bleeding associated with hormonal contraception. Am Fam Physician 2002;65:2073-2080.

Smith-Bindman R, Kerlikowske K, Feldstein VA : Endovaginal ultrasound to exclude endometrial cancer and other endometrial abnormalities. JAMA 1998;280:1510-1517.

Tabor A, Watt HC, Wald NJ: Endometrial thickness as a test for endometrial cancer in women with postmenopausal vaginal bleeding. Obstet Gynecol 2002;99:663-670.

30 POSTPARTUM DEPRESSION

Theodore O'Connell

According to the *Diagnostic and Statistical Manual of Mental Disorders*, 4th edition, major depression is defined by the presence of five of the following symptoms, one of which must be either depressed mood or decreased interest or pleasure in activities:

- Depressed mood, often accompanied or overshadowed by severe anxiety
- Markedly diminished interest or pleasure in activities
- Appetite disturbance: usually loss of appetite with weight loss
- Sleep disturbance: most often insomnia and fragmented sleep (in new mothers, even when the baby sleeps)
- Physical agitation (most commonly) or psychomotor slowing
- Fatigue and decreased energy
- Feelings of worthlessness or excessive or inappropriate guilt
- Decreased concentration or ability to make decisions
- Recurrent thoughts of death or suicidal ideation

The psychiatric postpartum experiences usually are divided into three categories: "maternal blues," postpartum depression, and postpartum psychosis.

"Maternal blues," also known as the "baby blues," is a transient state of heightened emotional reactivity that occurs in up to 85% of new mothers. Symptoms such as weeping, sadness, anxiety, irritability, and confusion occur, peaking around the 4th postpartum day and resolving by the 10th day.

Postpartum depression is a clinical term referring to a major depressive episode that is temporally associated with childbirth. An episode of depression is considered to have postpartum onset if it begins within 4 weeks after delivery. However, most investigators and clinicians use a time frame from 24 hours to 6 months after delivery to define postpartum depression. In fact, depressive episodes at any time within the first year after delivery may also be considered being postpartum in onset.

Postpartum depression occurs in approximately 10% to 20% of women in the United States within 6 months of delivery.

Postpartum psychosis occurs in 0.2% of childbearing women and usually begins during the first 4 weeks after delivery. The psychosis is typically manic in nature and in most cases may be considered a manifestation of bipolar disorder. Early warning signs include insomnia for several nights, agitation, an irritable or expansive mood, and avoidance of the infant. When delusions or hallucinations are present, they often involve the infant. Postpartum psychosis is considered a medical emergency because the affected woman is at risk for harming herself or her baby.

If the patient has considered a plan to act on suicidal thoughts or has thoughts about harming her infant, provisions for safety and urgent referral for psychiatric care are recommended.

The Edinburgh Postnatal Depression Scale (Table 30-1) is a 10-item questionnaire that is an effective screening tool for postpartum depression. A cutoff score of 9 or 10 has been recommended as a reliable indicator for the presence of postpartum depression in women in the United States. A clinical interview to review symptoms and establish the diagnosis of depression is warranted. A score between 5 and 9 should be evaluated again 2 to 4 weeks later in order to determine whether an episode of depression has evolved or whether symptoms have subsided.

Other postpartum depression screening tools include the Postpartum Depression Checklist, the Beck Depression Inventory, and the Center for Epidemiologic Studies Depression Scale.

Risk Factors for Postpartum Depression

Personal or family history of depression

Personal or family history of other psychiatric disease

History of premenstrual dysphoric disorder

Stressful life events

Marital discord

Inadequate social support

Suggested Work-Up

Thyroid-stimulating hormone (TSH) measurement	To evaluate for hypothyroidism or hyperthyroidism
Complete blood cell count (CBC)	To evaluate for anemia

Please circle the answer that best describes how you have felt over the past 7 days.

1. I have been able to laugh and see the funny side of things.
   0 = as much as I could
   1 = not quite so much now
   2 = definitely not so much now
   3 = not at all

2. I have looked forward with enjoyment to things.
   0 = as much as I ever did
   1 = rather less than I used to
   2 = definitely less than I used to do
   3 = hardly at all

3. I have blamed myself unnecessarily when things went wrong.
   3 = yes, most of the time
   2 = yes, sometimes
   1 = hardly ever
   0 = no, not at all

4. I have been anxious or worried for no good reason.
   3 = yes, very often
   2 = yes, sometimes
   1 = hardly ever
   0 = no, not at all

5. I have felt scared or panicky for no very good reason.
   3 = yes, quite a lot to me
   2 = yes, sometimes
   1 = no, not much
   0 = no, not at all

6. Things have been getting on top of me.
   3 = yes, most of the time I haven't been able to cope at all
   2 = yes, sometimes I haven't been coping as well as usual
   1 = no, most of the time I have coped quite well
   0 = no, I have been coping as well as ever

7. I have been so unhappy that I have had difficulty sleeping.
   3 = yes, most of the time
   2 = yes, sometimes
   1 = not very often
   0 = no, not at all

8. I have felt sad or miserable.
   3 = yes, most of the time
   2 = yes, quite often
   1 = not very often
   0 = no, not at all

9. I have been so unhappy that I have been crying.
   3 = yes, most of the time
   2 = yes, quite often
   1 = only occasionally
   0 = no, never

10. The thought of harming myself has occurred to me.
   3 = yes, quite often
   2 = sometimes
   1 = hardly ever
   0 = never

Table 30-1. Edinburgh Postnatal Depression Scale. *(From Cox JL, Holden JM, Sagovsky R: Detection of postnatal depression: development of the 10-item Edinburgh Postnatal Depression Scale. Br J Psychiatry 1987;150:782-786.)*

FURTHER READING

American Psychiatric Association: Diagnostic and Statistical Manual of Mental Disorders, 4th ed. Washington, DC: American Psychiatric Association, 1994.

Beck CT: Screening methods for postpartum depression. J Obstet Gynecol Neonatal Nurs 1995;24:308-312.

Brockington I: Postpartum psychiatric disorders. Lancet 2004;363:303-310.

Clay EC, Seehusen DA: A review of postpartum depression for the primary care physician. South Med J 2004;97:157-161.

Cox JL, Holden JM, Sagovsky R: Detection of postnatal depression: development of the 10-item Edinburgh Postnatal Depression Scale. Br J Psychiatry 1987;150:782-786.

Epperson CN: Postpartum major depression: detection and treatment. Am Fam Physician 1999;59:2247-2254.

Miller LJ: Postpartum depression. JAMA 2002;287:762-765.

Sharp LK, Lipsky MS: Screening for depression across the lifespan: a review of measures for use in primary care settings. Am Fam Physician 2002;66:1001-1008.

Wisner KL, Parry BL, Piontek CM: Postpartum depression. N Engl J Med 2002;347:194-199.

31 PRECOCIOUS PUBERTY

Theodore O'Connell

Normal puberty begins in girls between 8 and 14 years of age with breast buds and skeletal growth, followed by the arrival of pubic hair, axillary hair, and menarche. The age at which pubertal milestones are attained varies. In addition, it is influenced by activity level and nutritional status. Girls with low body fat may have a significant delay in menarche (up to a year or more), whereas obese girls may have earlier onset of puberty.

Precocious puberty is defined as the development of secondary sexual characteristics before the age of 8 years in girls. It involves not only early physical changes of puberty but also linear growth acceleration and acceleration of bone maturation, which leads to early epiphyseal fusion and short adult height.

There are two types of precocious puberty. Central precocious puberty results, or gonadotropin-releasing hormone (GnRH)—dependent precocious puberty, results from the premature activation of the hypothalamic GnRH pulse generator—pituitary gonadotropin—gonadal axis. In GnRH-independent precocious puberty, sex steroid secretion is independent of the GnRH pulse generator. Pathologic causes of puberty are likely if sexual development occurs in very young children or if there is contrasexual development. Peripheral causes are always pathologic and tend to produce an atypical puberty with loss of synchronicity of pubertal milestones.

Central precocious puberty is more common by far in girls than in boys, and in girls it is idiopathic in 95% of cases. In girls, therefore, additional investigation can be based on the clinical impression. Central nervous system (CNS) disorders account for a higher percentage of cases in boys but must also be investigated in girls.

Pubertal variants cause isolated development of one of the secondary sexual characteristics without accelerated skeletal maturation, and on occasion, they can progress to precocious puberty:

- *Simple premature thelarche* involves only breast development (unilateral or bilateral) without pubic hair growth, without accelerated bone maturation, and with a normal height outcome. No treatment is required. The disorder is usually self-limited and can resolve spontaneously or persist to normal puberty.

- *Simple premature adrenarche* involves only pubic hair development (pubic and axillary) without the other manifestations of puberty. No treatment is required, although the possibility of late-onset congenital adrenal hyperplasia should be investigated with a measurement of the serum 17α-hydroxyprogesterone level. There is an increased incidence of simple premature adrenarche in patients with CNS abnormalities.

Patients with precocious puberty and pubertal variants require an initial bone age as a baseline. In precocious puberty, the bone age is usually accelerated more than two standard deviations above the chronologic age. In pubertal variants, the bone age is within two standard deviations of the chronologic age. The bone age should be obtained at periodic intervals to determine whether pubertal variants have progressed to precocious puberty. The bone age is also used to monitor the effectiveness of therapy. Additional evaluation of precocious puberty is outlined below.

Medications Linked to Precocious Puberty

Androgens

Estrogens

Causes of Precocious Puberty

GnRH-Dependent Precocious Puberty

CNS tumors
- Astrocytoma
- Craniopharyngioma
- Ependymoma
- Hamartoma of the tuber cinereum
- Hypothalamic and optic gliomas
- Pinealoma

Previous CNS injury
- Cranial irradiation
- Head trauma
- Hypoxic-ischemic encephalopathy
- Infections (abscess, encephalitis, meningitis)

Other CNS disorders
- Arachnoid cyst
- Developmental abnormalities
- Hydrocephalus
- Neurofibromatosis type 1
- Sarcoid granuloma

- Septo-optic dysplasia
- Tuberculous granuloma
- Tuberous sclerosis

GnRH-Independent Precocious Puberty (in Girls)

Autonomously functioning ovarian cysts

Feminizing adrenal tumor

Hypothyroidism

Iatrogenic or exogenous sexual precocity

McCune-Albright syndrome

Ovarian tumors

- Carcinoma
- Cystadenoma
- Gonadoblastoma
- Granulosa-theca cell tumors
- Peutz-Jeghers syndrome

Key Historical Features

✓ Previous growth and development

✓ Sequence of pubertal events

✓ Medical history

✓ Surgical history

✓ Medications

✓ Detailed dietary history in underweight or overweight children

✓ Family history, especially history of genetic disease or precocious or delayed puberty

Key Physical Findings

✓ Vital signs

✓ Evaluation of growth chart

✓ Head and neck examination to evaluate the optic fundi, estimate the visual fields, and evaluate the sense of smell

✓ Determination of the Tanner stage of pubertal development

✓ Breast examination for pubertal development and asymmetry

✓ Genital examination for pubertal development

Suggested Work-Up

Radiograph of the left wrist	To estimate physiologic age for comparison with the child's chronologic age
Measurement of serum follicle-stimulating hormone (FSH), luteinizing hormone (LH), estradiol, testosterone, thyroid-stimulating hormone (TSH), thyroxine (T4), and human chorionic gonadotropin (hCG)	To confirm the impression of idiopathic precocious puberty, to localize the abnormality of the pathologic cause of precocious puberty, or to guide the choice of imaging study
Measurement of serum 17α-hydroxyprogesterone and dehydroepiandrosterone sulfate (DHEAS)	If a peripheral cause is suspected or if virilization is present in a female patient
Pelvic ultrasonography	To determine whether pubertal changes have occurred in the uterus and ovaries; also indicated if a peripheral cause (ovarian tumor) is suspected

Additional Work-Up

Magnetic resonance imaging (MRI) of the brain and pituitary gland	If a central pathologic cause is suspected on the basis of hormone measurements
GnRH stimulation test	Administration of 2.5 μg/kg of GnRH either intravenously or subcutaneously after an overnight fast; measurement of serum levels of FSH and LH at baseline just before the injection and 15, 30, 45, and 60 minutes after the injection
	Test interpretation is controversial, but a twofold to threefold rise in FSH and LH may observed if the patient has central precocious puberty; a peak LH level of more than 15 IU/L and a peak LH–to–peak FSH ratio of more than 0.66 are also criteria for defining a pubertal GnRH test result

Breast ultrasonography	Indicated in unilateral or asymmetric premature thelarche to rule out masses
Skeletal survey or radionuclide bone scan	Indicated for patients with McCune-Albright syndrome to evaluate for lesions of fibrous dysplasia

FURTHER READING

Bates GW: Hirsutism and androgen excess in childhood and adolescence, Pediatr Clin North Am 1981;28:513-530.

Blondell RD, Foster MB, Dave KC: Disorders of puberty, Am Fam Physician 1999;60: 209-224.

Fahmy JL, Kaminsky CK, Kaufman F, et al: The radiological approach to precocious puberty, Br J Radiol 2000;73:560-567.

Klein KO: Precocious puberty: who has it? Who should be treated?, J Clin Endocrinol Metab 1999;84:411-414.

Theodore O'Connell

Premenstrual syndrome (PMS) is characterized by the cyclic recurrence of symptoms during the luteal phase of the menstrual cycle. Premenstrual dysphoric disorder (PMDD) is a severe form of PMS. Of women of reproductive age, 80% have physical changes, such as breast tenderness or abdominal bloating, that are associated with menstruation; of these women, 20% to 40% experience symptoms of PMS, and 2% to 10% report severe disruption of their daily activities. The American College of Obstetrics and Gynecology (ACOG) recommends the PMS diagnostic criteria developed by the University of California at San Diego and the National Institute of Mental Health. These criteria are presented in Box 32-1.

PMDD is characterized by various combinations of marked mood swings, depressed mood, irritability, and anxiety, which may be accompanied by physical symptoms. These symptoms occur exclusively during the luteal phase of the menstrual cycle and generally resolve within 2 to 3 days after the onset of menses. The symptoms cause substantial impairment of personal functioning, generally more in social than occupational domains. A symptom-free period during the follicular phase of the menstrual cycle is essential in differentiating PMDD from preexisting anxiety or mood disorders.

Features of PMDD and depressive disorders overlap considerably. A family history of depression is common in women diagnosed with moderate to severe PMS. Despite the overlap between PMDD and depressive disorders, many patients with PMDD do not have depressive symptoms; therefore, PMDD should not be considered simply a variant of depressive disorder. The diagnostic criteria for PMDD from the *Diagnostic and Statistical Manual of Mental Disorders*, 4th edition, are presented in Box 32-2.

PMS and PMDD can be diagnosed only after physical and psychiatric disorders have been ruled out. This differential diagnosis is presented later in this chapter. PMS should be distinguished from simple premenstrual symptoms such as breast tenderness that does not interfere with daily functioning. The key elements of the diagnosis are symptoms consistent with PMS or PMDD, consistent occurrence of symptoms only during the luteal phase of the menstrual cycle, a relative absence of symptoms during the follicular phase of the menstrual cycle, and a negative impact of symptoms on function and lifestyle.

Medications Associated with Premenstrual Syndrome and Premenstrual Dysphoric Disorder

Oral contraceptives

National Institute of Mental Health

Both of the following criteria must be present:

- A 30% increase in the intensity of symptoms of premenstrual syndrome (measured on a standardized instrument) from cycle days 5 to 10 in comparison with the 6-day interval before the onset of menses

- Documentation of these changes in a daily symptom diary for at least two consecutive cycles

University of California at San Diego

At least one of the following affective and somatic symptoms occurs during the 5 days before menses in each of the three previous cycles:

- Affective symptoms: depression, angry outbursts, irritability, anxiety, confusion, social withdrawal

- Somatic symptoms: breast tenderness, abdominal bloating, headache, swelling of extremities

- Symptoms relieved from days 4 through 13 of the menstrual cycle

From American College of Obstetrics and Gynecology Practice Bulletin: Clinical management guidelines for obstetrician-gynecologists. Number 15, April 2000. Premenstrual syndrome. Obstet Gynecol 2000;95:1-9; and Kessel B: Premenstrual syndrome. Advances in diagnosis and treatment. Obstet Gynecol Clin North Am 2000;27:625-39.

Box 32-1. Diagnostic Criteria for Premenstrual Syndrome

Differential Diagnosis of Premenstrual Syndrome and Premenstrual Dysphoric Disorder

Affective disorder

- Anxiety
- Depression
- Dysthymia
- Panic disorder

Anemia

Anorexia

Bulimia

Chronic medical conditions such as diabetes

Dysmenorrhea

Endometriosis

Hypothyroidism

Oral contraceptive side effects

Perimenopause

Personality disorder

Substance abuse

A. In most menstrual cycles during the past year, five (or more) of the following symptoms were present for most of the time during the last week of the luteal phase, began to remit within a few days after the onset of the follicular phase, and were absent in the week after menses, with as least one of the symptoms being 1, 2, 3, or 4:

1. Markedly depressed mood, feelings of hopelessness, or self-deprecating thoughts

2. Marked anxiety, tension, or feelings of being "keyed up" or "on edge"

3. Marked affective lability (e.g., feeling suddenly sad or tearful or increased sensitivity to rejection)

4. Persistent and marked anger or irritability or increased interpersonal conflicts

5. Decreased interest in usual activities (e.g., work, school, friends, hobbies)

6. Subjective sense of difficulty in concentrating

7. Lethargy, easy fatigability, or marked lack of energy

8. Marked change in appetite, overeating, or specific food cravings

9. Hypersomnia or insomnia

10. A subjective sense of being overwhelmed or out of control

11. Other physical symptoms, such as breast tenderness or swelling, headaches, joint or muscle pain, a sensation of "bloating," or weight gain

B. The disturbance markedly interferes with work or school or with usual social activities and relationships with others (e.g., avoidance of social activities, decreased productivity and efficiency at work or school).

C. The disturbance is not merely an exacerbation of the symptoms of another disorder, such as major depressive disorder, panic disorder, dysthymic disorder, or a personality disorder (although it may be superimposed on any of these disorders).

D. Criteria A, B, and C must be confirmed by prospective daily ratings during at least two consecutive symptomatic cycles. (The diagnosis may be made provisionally before this confirmation.)

From American Psychiatric Association: Diagnostic and Statistical Manual of Mental Disorders, 4th ed. Washington, DC: American Psychiatric Association, 1994:717-718.

Box 32-2. Research Criteria for Premenstrual Dysphoric Disorder

Key Historical Features

✓ Duration of symptoms

✓ Interference with work, school, social activities, or relationships

✓ Affective or cognitive symptoms

- Affective lability (e.g., feeling suddenly sad or tearful or increased sensitivity to rejection)

- Aggression

- Anger
- Anxiety, tension, or feelings of being "keyed up" or "on edge"
- Decreased interest in usual activities (e.g., work, school, friends, hobbies)
- Depressed mood, feelings of hopelessness, or self-deprecating thoughts
- Fatigue
- Forgetfulness
- Hypersomnia or insomnia
- Irritability
- Panic attacks
- Poor concentration
- Reduced coping skills
- Subjective sense of difficulty in concentrating
- Marked change in appetite, overeating, or specific food cravings

✓ Other physical symptoms

- Acne
- Appetite change
- Bloating or fluid retention
- Breast tenderness or swelling
- Constipation
- Dizziness
- Fatigue
- Headaches
- Hot flashes
- Joint or muscle pain
- Muscle aches
- Nausea and vomiting
- Palpitations
- Pelvic heaviness or pressure
- Weight gain

✓ Medical history

✓ Surgical history

✓ Medications

✓ Family medical history

✓ Social history

Key Physical Findings

A comprehensive physical examination should be performed to rule out other possible causes of the emotional and physical symptoms.

Important considerations include a thyroid examination and a cardiopulmonary examination. The patient should be evaluated for evidence of alcohol or substance abuse and also for evidence of anorexia or bulimia.

Suggested Work-Up

The timing of symptoms should be confirmed with a prospective symptom and menstrual period record kept by the patient for at least two or three menstrual cycles. In the Daily Symptom Report, a self-reporting scale presented in Figure 32-1, patients rate each symptom on a 5-point scale from 0 (none) to 4 (severe). The scale provides guidance for scoring the severity of each symptom and may be used in the office setting for the diagnosis and assessment of PMDD.

For both PMS and PMDD, symptoms begin any time in the 2 weeks before the onset of menstrual flow, continue to the onset of menses, and resolve within 2 to 3 days after the onset of bleeding.

Diagnostic criteria for PMS and PMDD are outlined in Boxes 32-1 and 32-2.

A laboratory workup is not necessary unless the history or physical examination results are suggestive of physical or psychiatric disorders that could cause the patient's symptoms.

Additional Work-Up

Thyroid-stimulating hormone (TSH)	If a thyroid disorder is suspected
Complete blood cell count (CBC)	If anemia is suspected
Measurement of fasting blood glucose	If diabetes is suspected
Measurement of electrolytes, blood urea nitrogen (BUN), creatinine, calcium, magnesium, phosphorus, and albumin	If an eating disorder is suspected
Toxicology screen	If substance abuse is suspected
Abdominal ultrasonography, laparoscopy, or both	If endometriosis is suspected

Symptoms → / Days ↓	Anxiety	Irritability	Depression	Nervous tension	Mood swings	Feeling out of control	Poor coordination	Insomnia	Confusion	Headache	Crying	Fatigue	Aches	Breast tenderness	Cramps	Swelling	Food cravings	Daily Total Score
1																		
2																		
3																		
4																		
5																		
6																		
7																		
8																		
9																		
10																		
11																		
12																		
13																		
14																		
15																		
16																		
17																		
18																		
19																		
20																		
21																		
22																		
23																		
24																		
25																		
26																		
27																		
28																		
1																		

Severity scoring for each symptom:
0 = No symptom
1 = Minimal or slightly apparent to you
2 = Moderate, awareness of symptom but does not affect your daily routine
3 = A lot, continuously bothered by the symptom and/or symptoms interferes with your daily routine
4 = Severe, symptom is overwhelming and/or unable to carry out your daily routine

Day 1 is first day of menses

Figure 32-1. Daily symptom report. (From Freeman EW, DeRubeis RJ, Rickels K: Reliability and validity of a daily diary for premenstrual syndrome. Psychiatry Res 1996;65:97-106.)

FURTHER READING

ACOG Practice Bulletin: Clinical management guidelines for obstetrician-gynecologists. Number 15, April 2000. Premenstrual syndrome. Obstet Gynecol 2000;95:1-9.

American Psychiatric Association: Diagnostic and Statistical Manual of Mental Disorders, 4th ed. Washington, DC: American Psychiatric Association, 1994:717-718.

Bhatia SC, Bhatia SK: Diagnosis and treatment of premenstrual dysphoric disorder. Am Fam Physician 2002;66:1239-1248.

Dickerson LM, Mazyck PJ, Hunter MH: Premenstrual syndrome. Am Fam Physician 2003;67:1743-1752.

Freeman EW, DeRubeis RJ, Rickels K: Reliability and validity of a daily diary for premenstrual syndrome. Psychiatry Res 1996;65:97-106.

Frye GM, Silverman SD: Is it premenstrual syndrome? Keys to focused diagnosis, therapies for multiple symptoms. Postgrad Med 2000;107(5):151-154, 157-159.

Grady-Weliky TA: Premenstrual dysphoric disorder. N Engl J Med 2003;348:433-438.

Johnson SR: Premenstrual syndrome, premenstrual dysphoric disorder, and beyond: a clinical primer for practitioners. Obstet Gynecol 2004;104:845-859.

Kessel B: Premenstrual syndrome. Advances in diagnosis and treatment. Obstet Gynecol Clin North Am 2000;27:625-639.

Molin ML, Zendell SM: Evaluating and managing premenstrual syndrome. Medscape Womens Health 2000;5:1-16.

33 PRETERM LABOR

Theodore O'Connell

Preterm labor is the leading cause of perinatal morbidity and mortality in the United States. Preterm labor is characterized by increased uterine irritability and cervical effacement or dilatation, or both, before 37 weeks of pregnancy. Preterm labor usually results in preterm birth, which affects 8% to 10% of births in the United States. Unfortunately, in most cases, the precise causes of preterm labor are not known. Risk factors associated with preterm labor are outlined later in this chapter. Women with a history of preterm delivery have the highest risk of recurrence, estimated to be between 17% and 37%. Approximately 40% of spontaneous births following preterm labor are thought to be caused by infection. Screening and treatment for asymptomatic bacteriuria early in pregnancy, which prevents pyelonephritis during pregnancy, has helped reduce the rate of preterm delivery.

The identification of women with preterm contractions who will actually deliver before term is an inexact process. The inability to distinguish accurately between women in "true" preterm labor and those in "false" labor has hampered the assessment of therapeutic interventions, inasmuch as up to 50% of untreated patients do not actually deliver before term.

Several indicators have been studied as means of identifying women who will develop preterm labor and women who will deliver before term. Unfortunately, these indicators are imprecise markers of an activated process of parturition. Risk-scoring strategies have proved to be of limited value. Likewise, regular cervical assessment was found to have no predictive advantage in pregnant women with no predisposing risk factors. Although several studies have demonstrated an inverse relationship between cervix length and frequency of preterm delivery, transvaginal ultrasonography currently is not indicated in the routine evaluation of the patient with a history of or current risk factors for preterm delivery. Home monitoring of uterine activity may identify preterm contractions, but it is not clear whether the use of this system can affect the rate of preterm delivery.

Fetal fibronectin in cervical and vaginal secretions may be a biochemical marker for preterm labor. The presence of fetal fibronectin in the cervix or vagina is infrequent after the 20th week of gestation and rare after the 24th week. After the 24th week, the presence of fetal fibronectin may indicate detachment of the fetal membranes from the deciduas. Studies suggest that fetal fibronectin is a biochemical marker for labor. However, there is no evidence to suggest that the use of the assay for fetal fibronectin would result in a reduction in spontaneous preterm birth. Many questions still remain as to how to use the results of fetal fibronectin assays, both positive and negative, in clinical care.

Risk Factors for Preterm Labor

Abnormal placentation

Fetal causes

- Congenital anomalies
- Intrauterine fetal death
- Intrauterine growth retardation

Infectious causes

- Acute pyelonephritis
- Asymptomatic bacteriuria
- Bacterial vaginosis
- Cervical or vaginal colonization
- Chorioamnionitis

Low maternal body mass index

Low maternal socioeconomic status

Maternal age of less than 18 years or more than 40 years

Maternal complications

- Alcohol use
- Connective tissue disorders
- Gestational diabetes
- Illicit drug use
- Lack of prenatal care
- Periodontal infection
- Psychiatric disorders
- Pulmonary disease
- Short interpregnancy interval (<6 months)
- Smoking

Maternal history of one or more spontaneous second-trimester abortions

Multiple-fetus gestation

Nonwhite race

Nutritional deficiencies of copper and ascorbic acid

Presence of a retained intrauterine device

Preterm premature rupture of membranes

Previous preterm delivery

Uterine causes

- Amniocentesis
- Bicornate uterus
- Treatment for cervical incompetence, including conization or cerclage

- Exposure to diethylstilbestrol
- Myomata
- Uterine septum

Key Historical Features

✓ Gravity and parity

✓ Gestational age

✓ Frequency and duration of contractions

✓ Loss of fluid from the vagina

✓ Vaginal bleeding

✓ Abdominal pain

✓ Obstetric and gynecologic history

- Amniocentesis during current pregnancy
- History of previous preterm labor or preterm delivery
- History of cervical conization or cerclage
- Uterine septum or bicornate uterus

✓ Medical history

✓ Social history

- Smoking
- Alcohol use
- Illicit drug use
- Risk factors for sexually transmitted diseases

Key Physical Findings

✓ Vital signs

✓ Abdominal examination

✓ Sterile speculum examination to evaluate for cervical dilatation, vaginal bleeding, or infection and to determine whether rupture of amniotic membranes has occurred

✓ Determination of fetal presentation

✓ Determination of fetal station

Suggested Work-Up

Urine culture   Routine screening for asymptomatic bacteriuria, which should be performed at the initial prenatal visit; after therapy is

	completed, repeat of a urine culture to ensure eradication of infection
Tocodynamometry	To measure uterine activity
Sterile speculum examination	To evaluate for cervical dilatation, vaginal bleeding, or infection
Nitrazine test and fern test	To determine whether rupture of membranes has occurred
Measurement of fetal fibronectin obtained from vaginal fluid	May improve the diagnostic accuracy of preterm labor
Uterine ultrasonography	May be used alone or together with measurement of fetal fibronectin to try to diagnose preterm labor

Additional Work-Up

DNA test or culture for gonorrhea	Recommendations for routine screening vary: The Centers for Disease Control and Prevention (CDC) recommends that every pregnant woman undergo gonococcal screening at the initial visit; however, the American College of Gynecology and American Academy of Family Practice recommend screening only for patients with risk factors for gonorrhea
Urinalysis	If urinary tract infection is suspected
DNA test or culture for gonorrhea and chlamydia	If the patient has risk factors for infection or if physical examination suggests infection (mucopurulent cervical discharge and a hyperemic cervix)
Wet-mount examination, whiff test, and measurement of vaginal pH level	If bacterial vaginosis is suspected on examination (malodorous, thin discharge)
Wet-mount microscopy	If *Trichomonas* infection is suspected (copious yellow-gray homogenous discharge and an alkaline vaginal pH)

FURTHER READING

Ables AZ, Chauhan SP: Preterm labor: diagnostic and therapeutic options are not all alike. J Fam Pract 2005;54:245-252.

ACOG Committee on Practice Bulletins—Gynecology: ACOG Practice Bulletin No. 80: Premature rupture of membranes. Clinical management guidelines for obstetrician-gynecologists. Obstet Gynecol 2007;109:1007-1019.

Chatterjee J, Gullam J, Vatish M, et al: The management of preterm labour. Arch Dis Child Fetal Neonatal Ed 2007;92(2):F88-F93.

Cram LF, Zapata MI, Toy EC: Genitourinary infections and their association with preterm labor. Am Fam Physician 2002;65:241-248.

Goldenberg RL, Goepfert AR, Ramsey PS: Biochemical markers for the prediction of preterm birth. Am J Obstet Gynecol 2005;192(5 Suppl):S36-S46.

Simhan HN, Caritis SN: Prevention of preterm delivery. N Engl J Med 2007;357:477-487.

Weismiller DG: Preterm labor. Am Fam Physician 1999;57:2457-2464.

Theodore O'Connell

Miscarriage, or spontaneous abortion, is the spontaneous loss of a fetus at less than 20 weeks' gestation in the absence of elective medical or surgical measures to terminate the pregnancy. Recurrent miscarriage is defined as three or more consecutive pregnancy losses, although many clinicians define recurrent miscarriage as two or more losses. According to the latter definition, recurrent miscarriage affects from 1% to 5% of all couples trying to conceive. Fetal demise after the sixth month of gestation is rare, occurring in fewer than 4 per 1000 pregnancies.

Maternal age at conception is a strong independent risk factor for miscarriage, because of an increase in chromosomally abnormal conceptions. Reproductive history is also an independent predictor of future pregnancy outcome. Primigravidae and women with a history of live births have a lower risk of miscarriage in their next pregnancy than do women whose most recent pregnancy ended in miscarriage. Cigarette smoking, cocaine use, and alcohol use all increase the risk of miscarriage. Caffeine consumption is associated with a dose-dependent risk of miscarriage, which increases when intake exceeds 300 mg (three cups) of coffee daily.

Fetal aneuploidy is the most important cause of miscarriage before 10 weeks' gestation. At least 50% to 60% of all miscarriages are associated with cytogenetic abnormalities. Antiphospholipid syndrome is the most important treatable cause of recurrent miscarriage. Antiphospholipid antibodies, of which there are about 20, include lupus anticoagulant and anticardiolipin antibodies. The prevalence of antiphospholipid syndrome among women with recurrent miscarriage is 15%.

Causes of Recurrent Miscarriage

Endocrine causes

- Hyperprolactinemia
- Insulin resistance
- Polycystic ovary syndrome

Genetic and fetal causes

- Balanced reciprocal translocation
- Fetal aneuploidy, including trisomy, polyploidy, and monosomy X
- Congenital malformations

Immune causes (not conclusively proved)

- Maternal autoimmune disease

187

Infective causes

- Bacterial vaginosis
- Pathogens in the association of toxoplasmosis, other infections, rubella, cytomegalovirus infection, and herpes simplex (TORCH)

Rh incompatibility

Structural abnormalities

- Bicornate uterus
- Cervical incompetence
- Uterine fibroids (effect on reproductive outcome is controversial)
- Uterine septum

Thrombophilic disorders

- Acquired activated protein C resistance
- Antiphospholipid syndrome
- Antithrombin III deficiency
- Elevated factor VIII concentrations
- Factor V Leiden and activated protein C resistance
- Hyperhomocysteinemia
- Methylene tetrahydrofolate reductase C677T (MTHFR C677T)
- Protein C deficiency
- Protein S deficiency
- Prothrombin G20210A

Unexplained causes

Key Historical Features

✓ Obstetric and gynecologic history

- Menstrual history
- Previous pregnancies and their outcomes
- Previous pregnancy loss and timing of the loss
- Pelvic infections

✓ Medical history

✓ Surgical history

✓ Family history, especially history of recurrent miscarriage and genetic abnormalities

✓ Medications

Key Physical Findings

✓   General examination to evaluate for evidence of any systemic disease

✓   Pelvic examination to evaluate for uterine or adnexal abnormalities

Suggested Work-Up

Pelvic ultrasonography	To evaluate for uterine abnormalities and ovarian structure
Parental peripheral blood karyotype	To evaluate for an abnormal karyotype
Measurement of early follicular-phase follicle-stimulating hormone (FSH)	To assess ovarian reserve
Measurement of lupus anticoagulant antibody and anticardiolipin antibody	To evaluate for antiphospholipid syndrome
Test for Factor V Leiden	To evaluate for Factor V Leiden gene mutation
Test for prothrombin gene mutation	To evaluate for prothrombin G20210A gene mutation

Additional Work-Up

Measurement of protein S	If thrombophilia is suspected, to evaluate for protein S deficiency
Measurement of protein C	If thrombophilia is suspected, to evaluate for protein C deficiency
Measurement of antithrombin III	If thrombophilia is suspected, to evaluate for antithrombin deficiency
Measurement of homocysteine	If thrombophilia is suspected, to evaluate for hyperhomocysteinemia
Test for MTHFR C677T	If thrombophilia is suspected, to evaluate for point mutation in the methylene tetrahydrofolate reductase gene

FURTHER READING

Griebel CP, Halvorsen J, Golemon TB: Management of spontaneous abortion. Am Fam Physician 2005;72:1243-1250.

Hogge WA, Byrnes AL, Lanasa MC, et al: The clinical use of karyotyping spontaneous abortions. Am J Obstet Gynecol 2003;189:397-400.

Kujovich JL: Thrombophilia and pregnancy complications. Am J Obstet Gynecol 2004;191:412-424.

Miller TE, Estrella E, Myerburg RJ, et al: Recurrent third-trimester fetal loss and maternal mosaicism for long-QT syndrome. Circulation 2004;109:3029-3034.

Rai R, Regan L: Recurrent miscarriage. Lancet 2006;368:601-611.

Rasch V: Cigarette, alcohol and caffeine consumption: risk factors for spontaneous abortion. Acta Obstet Gynecol Scand 2003;82:182-188.

Walker ID: Thrombophilia in pregnancy. J Clin Pathol 2000;53:573-580.

Theodore O'Connell

In the general population, urinary tract infection (UTI) is primarily an infection of sexually active women; the prevalence of UTI in women outnumbers that in men by a ratio of 30:1. However, the prevalence of UTI increases in both sexes with advancing age, reducing the ratio to 2:1. Recurrent UTI is defined as three or more episodes of symptomatic bacteriuria within 1 year. A recurrent infection is one that occurs after documented, successful resolution of an antecedent infection.

In younger adults, recurrent infection occurs most often as a bladder infection in women and is usually related to sexual intercourse. In older persons, recurrence is primarily a lower tract disease as a result of different risk or contributing factors, which may include incomplete bladder emptying or diseases such as diabetes mellitus.

The decision to evaluate recurrent UTI radiologically, endoscopically, urodynamically, or otherwise should be based on the patient's clinical presentation, history, findings, response to antimicrobial therapy, and pattern of recurrent UTIs. Severe UTI—defined as sepsis, fever, history of UTI lasting more than 7 days, gross hematuria, signs or symptoms of obstruction, or history of stones—warrants further evaluation. Risk factors such as diabetes mellitus, immunosuppression, debilitating disease, or pregnancy also may warrant further evaluation.

If a patient has a history of recurrent UTI, urine culture should be used to document the infection, identify the pathogen, and determine the frequency of infection. Urine culture is also used to distinguish between unresolved and recurrent infection. If the same pathogen is documented repeatedly and at close intervals, an underlying abnormality should be suspected, and an evaluation should be initiated. If the same pathogen is not found or if UTIs do not occur in a close temporal relationship, the likelihood that the infections are associated with functional, metabolic, or anatomic abnormalities is low, and the patient may be treated with low-dose antimicrobial prophylaxis.

Conditions Associated with Recurrent Urinary Tract Infection

Advancing age

Bacterial resistance

Diabetes mellitus

Genitourinary anatomic abnormalities (bladder polyp, urethral diverticula, fistula, medullary sponge kidney)

Genitourinary calculi

Immunosuppression

Incomplete bladder emptying (spinal cord injury, neurogenic bladder, advancing age)

Indwelling catheter

Noncompliance with medication regimen

Perinephric abscess

Pregnancy

Pyelonephritis

Poor hygiene

Renal abscess

Sexual intercourse

Urinary diversion procedure

Urologic instrumentation

Key Historical Features

✓ Age

✓ Previous response to therapy and culture results

✓ Presence of fever, nausea, or malaise

✓ Frequency of infection and temporal relationship to intercourse

✓ Contraceptive practices

✓ Dysuria

✓ Urinary frequency

✓ Urgency

✓ Hematuria

✓ Vaginal discharge

✓ Odor

✓ Dyspareunia

✓ Pruritis

✓ History of childhood infections

✓ Medical history, especially history of urolithiasis, known urinary tract abnormality, immunosuppression, or diabetes mellitus

✓ Previous urologic surgery or instrumentation

Key Physical Findings

✓   Vital signs

✓   General examination to evaluate patient's overall health

✓   Abdominal examination

✓   Back examination to evaluate for costovertebral angle tenderness

✓   Genitourinary examination to evaluate for urethritis or vaginitis

✓   Gynecologic examination to rule out vaginal pathologic processes

Suggested Work-Up

Urinalysis	To determine whether the urine contains infectious organisms
Urine culture	To document infection, identify the pathogen, and determine the frequency of infection
Measurement of blood urea nitrogen (BUN) and creatinine	To evaluate renal function
Quantification of postvoid residual bladder volume	To evaluate bladder emptying

One of the following tests should be considered as well:

Renal ultrasonography	To evaluate upper urinary tract architecture and establish the presence of hydronephrosis or abscess
Intravenous pyelography	To evaluate for filling defects or diagnose obstructive uropathy
Computed tomographic (CT) scan	To evaluate anatomic detail and to diagnose the presence of urinary stones

Additional Work-Up

Voiding cystography	If an anatomic abnormality is suspected
Cystoscopy	If tumor or mass is suspected
Urology consultation	For obstructive uropathy, calculi, abscess, or genitourinary abnormalities

FURTHER READING

Engel JD, Schaeffer AJ: Evaluation of and antimicrobial therapy for recurrent urinary tract infections in women. Urol Clin North Am 1998;25:685-701.

McLaughlin SP, Carson CC: Urinary tract infections in women. Med Clin North Am 2004;88:417-429.

Pewitt EB, Schaeffer AJ: Urinary tract infection in urology, including acute and chronic prostatitis. Infect Dis Clin North Am 1997;11:623-646.

Yoshikawa TT, Nicolle LE, Norman DC: Management of complicated urinary tract infection in older patients. J Am Geriatr Soc 1996;44:1235-1241.

36 FEMALE SEXUAL DYSFUNCTION: DYSFUNCTION OF SEXUAL DESIRE, AROUSAL, AND ORGASM

Kathleen Dor

Problems with sexual desire, arousal, and orgasm in women are very common and cause significant personal distress. The American Foundation for Urologic Disease classifies these problems as four disorders: hypoactive sexual desire disorder, sexual aversion disorder, sexual arousal disorder, and female orgasmic disorder. A discussion of each of these disorders is beyond the scope of this text. Dyspareunia is discussed in Chapter 11.

A wide variety of factors contribute to sexual dysfunction, including age, smoking, chronic diseases, relationship difficulties, prior trauma, surgery, low socioeconomic status, and education. Individually, sexuality incorporates family, societal, and religious beliefs and is altered with aging, health status, and personal experience. Sexual activity also incorporates interpersonal relationships; each partner brings unique attitudes, needs, responses, and health matters into the sexual experience.

The diagnosis of female sexual dysfunction requires the physician to obtain a detailed patient history that defines the dysfunction, identifies causative or confounding medical or gynecologic problems, and contains pertinent psychosocial information. Establishment of the patient's sexual orientation is necessary and is best achieved through nonjudgmental, direct questions. Questioning the patient about what she thinks is causing the problem may elicit insight.

Medications That May Cause Sexual Dysfunction in Women

α-Adrenergic blockers

Amphetamines

Antiepileptic medications

Anticholinergic medications

Antipsychotic medications

Antihistamines

Benzodiazepines

β blockers

Cholesterol-lowering medications

Cyclophosphamide

Digitalis

Diuretics

Gonadotropin-releasing hormone agonists

Oral contraceptives

Selective serotonin reuptake inhibitors

Spironolactone

Trazodone

Vasodilators

Causes of Sexual Dysfunction (in Arousal, Desire, and Orgasm) in Women

Adrenal disorders

Aging

Alcohol overuse or abuse

Anxiety

Autoimmune diseases

Bowel incontinence

Breast cancer

Cardiac disease

Colostomy

Depression

Diabetes

Dyspareunia

Genital abnormalities

Gynecologic neoplasms

Gynecologic surgery

Hyperprolactinemia

Inadequate lubrication

Kidney failure

Liver failure

Lung disease

Medications

Menopause

Multiple sclerosis

Musculoskeletal diseases

Parkinson disease

Peripheral vascular disease

Relationship problems

Sexual or physical abuse

Spinal cord injury

Stress

Stroke

Testosterone deficiency

Urinary incontinence

Vaginal atrophy

Key Historical Features

✓ Symptoms of systemic disease

- Weakness
- Numbness
- Angina
- Shortness of breath
- Musculoskeletal pain or stiffness
- Claudication
- Fatigue

✓ Medical history

- Especially a history of diabetes, breast cancer, gynecologic cancers, cardiovascular disease, neurologic diseases, musculoskeletal diseases, endocrinologic diseases, use of urinary catheters, or colostomies

✓ Psychiatric history

- Symptoms of or a prior diagnosis of depression or anxiety, which can cause sexual dysfunction (psychiatric illness can also be exacerbated by sexual dysfunction)

✓ Medications

✓ History of recreational drug use

- Alcohol, tobacco, or illicit drug use, which can be risk factors for sexual dysfunction

✓ Obstetric/gynecologic history

- Obstetric history, especially prior surgical deliveries and trauma during deliveries
- History of surgery, endometriosis, prolapse, urinary incontinence, and pelvic trauma (including motor vehicle accidents)

✓ Sexual history (consider using a validated index, such as the Female Sexual Function questionnaire)

- Prior sexual experience
- Sexual orientation
- Nature of the problem
- Onset and duration of the problem
- Partner's response to problem
- Response to masturbation
- History of sexual abuse

Key Physical Findings

✓ Vital signs

✓ General appearance

✓ Neck examination to evaluate for thyroid nodules or a goiter

✓ Cardiovascular examination to evaluate for murmurs, abnormal heart sounds, and peripheral pulses

✓ Pulmonary examination to evaluate for crackles or wheezes

✓ Musculoskeletal examination to evaluate for disabilities that could interfere with sexual function

✓ Neurologic examination to evaluate evidence of weakness, numbness, or abnormal reflexes

✓ Gynecologic examination

- Examination of the external genitalia for any lesions, atrophy, tenderness, or potentially embarrassing abnormalities (such as labial asymmetry); also, evaluation of amount of pubic hair, a decrease of which may indicate androgen deficiency

- Single-finger vaginal examination to palpate the walls of the vagina, as well as the bladder and urethra; evaluation of the tone of the pelvic floor muscles and voluntary muscle control; and assessment for cystocele, rectocele, or uterine prolapse, which may result in incontinence and in avoidance of sexual relations

- Speculum examination with a narrow speculum that is lubricated, to examine the vaginal mucosa and cervix

- Bimanual examination to evaluate for cervical motion tenderness, adnexal or uterine tenderness, or any masses or nodules

Suggested Work-Up

Measurement of follicle-stimulating hormone (FSH) and luteinizing hormone (LH)	To evaluate for hormonal imbalance and menopausal status
Measurement of thyroid-stimulating hormone (TSH)	To evaluate for thyroid disease
Measurement of prolactin level	To evaluate for hyperprolactinemia
Measurement of serum estradiol	To evaluate for estrogen deficiency
Measurements of total and free testosterone	To evaluate for testosterone deficiency
Measurement of fasting blood glucose	To evaluate for diabetes

Additional Work-Up

Measurement of dehydroepiandrosterone sulfate (DHEAS)	To evaluate for adrenal hyperplasia
Complete blood cell count	To evaluate for anemia
Liver function tests	If liver disease or liver failure is suspected
Measurement of blood urea nitrogen (BUN) and creatinine	If renal failure is suspected

FURTHER READING

Basson R: Sexual desire and arousal disorders in women. N Engl J Med 2006;354:1497-1506.

Carey JC: Pharmacological effects on sexual function. Obstet Gynecol Clin North Am 2006;22:599-620.

Drugs that cause sexual dysfunction: an update. Med Lett Drugs Ther 1992;34(876):73-78.

Lightner DJ: Female sexual dysfunction. Mayo Clin Proc 2002;77:698-702.

Pauls RN, Kleeman SD, Karram MM: Female sexual dysfunction: principles of diagnosis and therapy. Obstet Gynecol Surv 2005;60(3):196-205.

Phillips NA: Female sexual dysfunction: evaluation and treatment. Am Fam Physician 2000;62:127-136.

37 URINARY INCONTINENCE

Theodore O'Connell

Urinary incontinence is caused by disturbance in the storage function, and occasionally in the emptying function, of the lower urinary tract. A continent sphincter mechanism requires proper angulation between the urethra and the bladder, as well as proper positioning of the urethra so that increases in intra-abdominal pressure are effectively transmitted to the urethra.

Women may undergo an anatomic or neuromuscular injury during childbirth but remain clinically asymptomatic as long as there is compensation by other components of the continence mechanism. Incontinence may not manifest in a woman until she loses a small percentage of muscle strength and innervation in the urethral sphincter as a result of aging or other injuries.

Stress incontinence is the involuntary loss of urine during an increase of intra-abdominal pressure. Stress urinary incontinence arises when bladder pressure exceeds urethral pressure during activities such as coughing, laughing, or exercising. The underlying abnormality is typically urethral hypermobility caused by a failure of the normal anatomic supports of the bladder neck. Intrinsic urethral sphincter deficiency, the lack of normal intrinsic pressure within the urethra, may also lead to stress incontinence.

Overactive bladder, also known as urge incontinence, is the involuntary loss of urine preceded by a strong urge to void regardless of whether the bladder is full. Urge incontinence results from bladder contractions that overwhelm the ability of the cerebral centers to inhibit them. This bladder oversensitivity may originate from the bladder epithelium or detrusor muscle as the result of altered neural activation in the voiding cycle.

Overflow incontinence is urine loss associated with overdistension of the bladder, typically caused by an underactive detrusor muscle, outlet obstruction, or both. Patients may have frequent or constant dribbling, overactive bladder, or stress incontinence. Causes of detrusor muscle underactivity are outlined later in this chapter. Overflow incontinence is relatively uncommon but is more common in men because of the prevalence of obstructive prostate gland enlargement.

The first goal of the evaluation of urinary incontinence is to identify reversible causes of incontinence so that effective treatments may be instituted. The second goal is to identify conditions that may necessitate special evaluation or referral to a urologist or urogynecologist. Once transient causes and indications for specialty evaluation or referral have been excluded, the third goal is to decide whether the patient's symptoms are more suggestive of urge incontinence or stress incontinence. After this has been determined, treatment may be initiated accordingly. If the treatment is ineffective, specialty evaluation may be indicated.

Indications for specialty evaluation or referral that are detected from history include recent onset within 2 months of urge incontinence or irritative bladder symptoms, previous surgery for incontinence, previous radical pelvic surgery, or incontinence associated with recurrent symptomatic urinary infections. Physical findings that usually necessitate specialty referral include gross pelvic prolapse and neurologic abnormalities suggestive of a systemic disorder or spinal cord lesion. Hematuria without infection and significant persistent proteinuria on urinalysis necessitate additional evaluation. Other situations that may necessitate specialty evaluation or referral are an abnormal postvoid residual volume, treatment failure, consideration of surgical intervention, or an inability to establish a presumptive diagnosis and treatment plan.

Medications Linked to Urinary Incontinence

α-Adrenergic agonists

α-Adrenergic blockers

Angiotensin-converting enzyme (ACE) inhibitors

Anticholinergic agents

Antidepressants

Antihistamines

Antipsychotics

β Blockers

Calcium channel blockers

Diuretics

Lithium

Narcotics

Sedatives

Causes of Urinary Incontinence

Overflow incontinence

- Diabetic neuropathy
- Fecal impaction
- Medications
- Radiation
- Tumor
- Surgery
- Urethral stricture

Stress incontinence

- Intrinsic sphincter deficiency
- Medications

- Pelvic prolapse
- Radiation damage
- Surgical trauma
- Urethral hypermobility

Urge incontinence

- Alcohol
- Atrophic vaginitis
- Caffeine
- Calculi
- Dementia
- Encephalopathy
- Hypoxemia
- Impaired mobility
- Infection
- Malignancy
- Medications
- Parkinson disease
- Stroke

Key Historical Features

✓ Frequency of episodes

✓ Degree of bother to the patient

✓ Leakage of urine

- With coughing, laughing, lifting, or sneezing
- In association with a strong urge to urinate
- During sex
- Without the patient's being aware of the leakage

✓ Use of pad to protect clothing from leaking urine

✓ Time of day or night

✓ Relation to medication treatments

✓ Fluid intake

✓ Voiding habits

✓ How often sleep is interrupted by the need to urinate

✓ Presence of dysuria

✓ Sensation of incomplete bladder emptying

✓ Frequency of bowel movements

✓ Splinting of the vagina or perineum during defecation

✓ Presence of fecal incontinence

✓ Medical history

- Chronic lung disease
- Cognitive impairment
- Diabetes
- Fecal impaction
- Lumbar disk disease
- Stroke

✓ Obstetric and gynecologic history

- Gravity and parity
- Number of vaginal, instrument-assisted, and cesarean deliveries
- Estrogen status
- Time interval between deliveries
- Hysterectomy, vaginal surgery
- Bladder surgery
- Pelvic trauma
- Pelvic radiotherapy

✓ Surgical history

✓ Medications

Key Physical Findings

✓ General examination for mobility status

✓ Neurologic examination for cognitive status, upper motor neuron lesions such as multiple sclerosis or Parkinson disease, lower motor neuron lesions such as sacral-nerve root lesions; assessment of lumbosacral nerve roots by checking deep tendon reflexes, lower extremity strength, and sharp or dull sensation

✓ Cardiovascular and pulmonary examination to assess for causes of cough

✓ Abdominal examination for masses, diastasis recti abdominis, ascites, or organomegaly

✓ Pelvic examination for pelvic masses, organ prolapse, or vaginal atrophy (the levator ani muscle function can be evaluated by asking the patient to tighten her vaginal muscles and hold the contraction as long as possible); evaluation of the bulbocavernous and clitoral sacral reflexes; and evaluation for inflammation, infection, and atrophy

✓ Rectal examination to evaluate for sphincter tone, fecal impaction, rectal lesions, or the presence of occult blood

✓ Extremity examination for peripheral edema

✓ Urine leakage should be assessed with coughing or Valsalva maneuver in both the supine and standing position

Suggested Work-Up

Urinalysis	To evaluate for urinary tract infection or diabetes-induced glycosuria
Urine culture	Not routinely indicated but possibly useful in identifying the causative organism of infections and in guiding antibiotic therapy
Assessment of postvoid residual volume by catheterization or ultrasonography	To detect urinary retention (<50 mL is normal; >200 mL is abnormal).
Cystometry	To measure bladder pressure during filling, which provides information about bladder capacity and the ability to inhibit detrusor contractions
Cystoscopy	Indicated for the evaluation of patients with incontinence who also have any of the following: hematuria or pyuria; irritative voiding symptoms such as frequency, urgency, and urge incontinence in the absence of reversible causes; bladder pain; recurrent cystitis; and suburethral mass
	Also indicated when urodynamic testing fails to duplicate symptoms of urinary incontinence

Additional Work-Up

Cystometric testing	Indicated as part of the evaluation of more complex disorders of bladder filling and voiding, such as the presence of neurologic disease and

	other comorbid conditions (there is only limited data suggestive of its need in the routine evaluation of women with urinary incontinence)
Urodynamic testing	May be indicated when surgical treatment of stress incontinence is planned
Pressure-flow voiding studies, uroflowmetry, and electromyography of the anal sphincter	May be indicated for the assessment of complex and neurogenic causes of urinary incontinence and voiding disorders

FURTHER READING

Culligan PJ, Heit M: Urinary incontinence in women: evaluation and management. Am Fam Physician 2000;62:2433-2444.

Morantz CA: ACOG guidelines on urinary incontinence in women. Am Fam Physician 2005;72:175.

Norton P, Brubaker L: Urinary incontinence in women. Lancet 2006;367:57-67.

Wein AJ, Rackley RR: Overactive bladder: a better understanding of pathophysiology, diagnosis, and management. J Urol 2006;175:S5-S10.

Weiss BD: Diagnostic evaluation of urinary incontinence in geriatric patients. Am Fam Physician 1998;57:2675-2684.

38 VACCINATIONS DURING PREGNANCY

Theodore O'Connell

The administration of vaccines during pregnancy often poses concerns to physicians and patients about the risk of transmitting a virus to a developing fetus (Tables 38-1 and 38-2). However, for a developing fetus, this risk from vaccination of the mother during pregnancy is theoretical. There is no evidence of risk from vaccinating pregnant women with inactivated viral or bacterial vaccines or toxoids.

Live-virus vaccines, however, do pose a theoretical risk to the fetus. In general, live-virus vaccines are contraindicated in pregnant women because of the theoretical risk of transmission of the vaccine virus to the fetus. If a live-virus vaccine is inadvertently given to a pregnant woman, or if a woman becomes pregnant within 4 weeks after vaccination, she should be counseled about the potential effects on the fetus. Such vaccination is not ordinarily an indication to terminate the pregnancy.

Vaccine	Should Be Considered if Otherwise Indicated	Contraindicated During Pregnancy	Special or Conditional Recommendation
Hepatitis A virus	X		The risk associated with vaccination should be weighed against the risk for hepatitis A in pregnant women who may be at high risk for exposure to hepatitis A virus
Hepatitis B virus	X		
Human papillomavirus (HPV)			Quadrivalent HPV vaccine is not recommended for use in pregnancy The vaccine has not been causally associated with adverse outcomes of pregnancy or adverse events to the developing fetus; however, data on vaccination during pregnancy are limited Until additional information becomes available, initiation of the vaccine series should be delayed until after completion of the pregnancy If a woman is found to be pregnant after initiating the vaccination series, the remainder of the three-dose regimen should be delayed until after completion of the pregnancy If a vaccine dose has been administered during pregnancy, no intervention is needed
Influenza virus (inactivated)	Recommended		
Influenza virus*		X	
Measles virus*		X	
Meningococcal virus (MCV4)			No data are available on the safety of MCV4 during pregnancy Women of childbearing age who become aware that they were pregnant at the time of MCV4 vaccination should contact their health care provider or the vaccine manufacturer
Mumps virus*		X	
Pneumococcal			The safety of pneumococcal polysaccharide vaccine during the first trimester of pregnancy has not been evaluated, although no adverse consequences have been reported among newborns whose mothers were inadvertently vaccinated during pregnancy
Polio virus (IPV)			Although no adverse effects of IPV have been documented among pregnant women or their fetuses, vaccination of pregnant women should be avoided on theoretical grounds; however, if a pregnant woman is at increased risk for infection and requires immediate protection against polio, IPV can be administered in accordance with the recommended schedule for adults

Continued

Table 38-1. Routine Vaccines

Vaccine	Should Be Considered if Otherwise Indicated	Contraindicated During Pregnancy	Special or Conditional Recommendation
Rubella virus*		X	
Tetanus-diphtheria (Td)	X		
Tetanus-diphtheria-pertussis (Tdap)			Pregnancy is not a contraindication for use of Tdap; Td is recommended when tetanus and diphtheria protection is required during pregnancy In some situations, health care providers can choose to administer Tdap instead of Td to add protection against pertussis When Td to Tdap is administered during pregnancy, the second or third trimester is preferred
Varicella virus		X	

Adapted from Guidelines for Vaccinating Pregnant Women. Recommendations of the Advisory Committee on Immunization Practices (ACIP), Atlanta, GA: Centers for Disease Control and Prevention, 2007.

*Live attenuated vaccine.

Table 38-1. Routine Vaccines

Vaccine	Should Be Considered if Otherwise Indicated	Contraindicated During Pregnancy	Special or Conditional Recommendation
Anthrax			Pregnant women should be vaccinated against anthrax only if the potential benefits of vaccination outweigh the potential risks to the fetus
Bacille Calmette-Guérin (BCG*)		×	
Japanese encephalitis			Japanese encephalitis vaccine should not be routinely administered during pregnancy Pregnant women who must travel to an area where risk of Japanese encephalitis is high should be vaccinated when the theoretical risks of immunization are outweighed by the risk of infection to the mother and developing fetus
Meningococcal virus (MPSV4)	×		
Rabies	×		
Typhoid (parenteral and oral*)			No data have been reported on the use of any of the three typhoid vaccines among pregnant women
Vaccinia virus*		×	Vaccinia vaccine should not be administered to pregnant women for routine nonemergency indications Pregnant women who have had a definite exposure to smallpox virus should be vaccinated
Yellow fever virus*			Yellow fever vaccine should be administered only if travel to an endemic area is unavoidable and if an increased risk for exposure exists
Zoster virus*		×	

Adapted from Guidelines for Vaccinating Pregnant Women. Recommendations of the Advisory Committee on Immunization Practices (ACIP). Atlanta, GA: Centers for Disease Control and Prevention, 2007.

*Live attenuated vaccine.

Table 39-2. Travel and Other Vaccines

FURTHER READING

Advisory Committee on Immunization Practices: Use of anthrax vaccine in the United States. MMWR Recomm Rep 2000;49(No. RR-15):1-20.

Bilukha OO, Rosenstein N, National Center for Infectious Diseases, Centers for Disease Control and Prevention: Prevention and control of meningococcal disease: recommendations of the Advisory Committee on Immunization Practices (ACIP). MMWR Recomm Rep 2005;54(No. RR-7):1-21.

Centers for Disease Control and Prevention: Prevention of Tetanus, Diphtheria and Pertussis Among Pregnant Women: Provisional ACIP Recommendations for the Use of Tdap Vaccine, 2006. Available at http://www.cdc.gov/nip/recs/provisional_recs/tdap-preg.pdf; accessed February 24, 2008.)

Cetron MS, Marfin AA, Julian KG, et al: Yellow fever vaccine: recommendations of the Advisory Committee on Immunization Practices (ACIP), 2002. MMWR 2002;51(No. RR-17):1-11.

Guidelines for Vaccinating Pregnant Women. Recommendations of the Advisory Committee on Immunization Practices (ACIP). Atlanta, GA: Centers for Disease Control and Prevention, 2007.

Inactivated Japanese encephalitis virus vaccine: recommendations of the Advisory Committee on Immunization Practices (ACIP). MMWR Recomm Rep 1993;42(No. RR-1):1-15.

Kroger AT, Atkinson WL, Marcuse EK, et al: General recommendations on immunization: recommendations of the Advisory Committee on Immunization Practices (ACIP). MMWR Recomm Rep 2006;55(No. RR-15):1-48.

Markowitz LE, Dunne EF, Saraiya M, et al: Quadrivalent human papillomavirus vaccine: recommendations of the Advisory Committee on Immunization Practices (ACIP). MMWR Recomm Rep 2007;56(No. RR-2):1-24.

Prevention of pneumococcal disease: recommendations of the Advisory Committee on Immunization Practices (ACIP). MMWR Recomm Rep 1997;46(No. RR-8):1-24.

Prevots DR, Burr RK, Sutter RW, et al: Poliomyelitis prevention in the United States: updated recommendations of the Advisory Committee on Immunization Practices (ACIP). MMWR Recomm Rep 2000;49(No. RR-5):1-22.

Rotz LD, Dotson DA, Damon IK, et al: Vaccinia (smallpox) vaccine: recommendations of the Advisory Committee on Immunization Practices (ACIP). MMWR Recomm Rep 2001;50(No. RR-10):1-25.

Sur DK, Wallis DH, O'Connell TX: Vaccinations in pregnancy. Am Fam Physician 2003;68:E299-E309.

Typhoid immunization. Recommendations of the Advisory Committee on Immunization Practices (ACIP). MMWR Recomm Rep 1990;39(No. RR-10):1-5.

39 VAGINAL BLEEDING IN EARLY PREGNANCY

Kathleen Dor

Vaginal bleeding in early pregnancy is common. The main differential diagnosis is threatened abortion, spontaneous abortion, ectopic pregnancy, and molar pregnancy.

Vaginal bleeding during early pregnancy is presumptively called a *threatened abortion* unless another cause is found. A threatened abortion occurs in 25% of all pregnancies and represents bleeding in the first trimester without passage of tissue. Half of all threatened abortions progress to a spontaneous abortion. However, only 4% to 10% of pregnancies with fetal cardiac activity and vaginal bleeding progress to a spontaneous abortion. Other related terms include *inevitable abortion* (rupture of membranes and/or cervical dilation during early pregnancy so that pregnancy loss is inevitable), *incomplete abortion* (only partial expulsion of products of conception occur), and *missed abortion* (retention of a failed pregnancy).

Ectopic pregnancy occurs in nearly 2% of pregnancies. Because life-threatening bleeding can occur, it is an important diagnosis to make. Risk factors include a history of salpingitis, previous ectopic pregnancy, and advanced maternal age.

Hydatidiform moles are caused by abnormal growth of the placental trophoblastic tissue. With a complete mole, a fetus does not develop. With a partial mole, an abnormal fetus develops. Hydatidiform moles can become malignant and develop into choriocarcinoma.

When a pregnant patient has vaginal bleeding in early pregnancy, a complete history and physical examination are important to determine the cause. The important elements are outlined as follows.

Medications Linked to Bleeding in Pregnancy

Aspirin

Clopidogrel

Heparin

Nonsteroidal anti-inflammatory drugs (NSAIDs)

Methotrexate

Misoprostol

Retinoids

Warfarin

Causes of Vaginal Bleeding in Early Pregnancy

Cervical disease
- Cervical cancer
- Cervical erosion
- Cervical polyps
- Cervical trauma
- Cervicitis

Ectopic pregnancy

Hematologic disorders
- Idiopathic thrombocytopenic purpura
- Leukemia
- von Willebrand disease

Induced abortion

Medications

Spontaneous abortion

Subchorionic bleeding

Threatened abortion

Trophoblastic disease
- Choriocarcinoma
- Hydatidiform mole

Vaginal disease
- Vaginal trauma
- Vaginitis

Key Historical Features

✓ Associated symptoms
- Fever, chills, or night sweats, which may indicate infection
- Dizziness, which may indicate a large amount of blood loss

✓ History of trauma

✓ Obstetric and gynecologic history
- Nature and amount of bleeding and passage of any tissue or clots
- Menstrual history
- Previous pregnancies and any complications, including prior spontaneous abortion
- Previous ultrasound examinations during this pregnancy and whether a viable intrauterine pregnancy was documented

- • Associated pelvic or abdominal pain, which may indicate ectopic pregnancy
- • Sexual history
- • History of any gynecologic surgery or procedures, especially recent procedures, including induced abortions
- • History of any sexually transmitted diseases or pelvic inflammatory disease

✓ Medical history, especially history of bleeding disorders

✓ Surgical history

✓ Family history

Key Physical Findings

✓ Vital signs, including orthostatic assessments

✓ Evidence of a bleeding disorder, such as bruising

✓ Gynecologic/obstetric examination

- • Perineum and vulvar examination for any lesions or trauma
- • Speculum examination to evaluate for any bleeding or cervical lesions and to determine whether the cervical os is open or closed
- • Bimanual examination to evaluate the size and consistency of the uterus and whether there is any uterine tenderness; in addition, evaluation for adnexal tenderness or masses (patients with a molar pregnancy often have a discrepancy between the uterine size and dates; patients with an ectopic pregnancy may have cervical motion tenderness or pelvic tenderness)

✓ Abdominal examination for tenderness, rebound, or guarding (the presence of peritoneal signs is suspect for ectopic pregnancy)

✓ Rectal examination to note the presence of any hemorrhoids

Suggested Work-Up

The key to evaluating vaginal bleeding in early pregnancy is to initially rule out ectopic pregnancy, especially if the patient is experiencing abdominal pain.

Urine pregnancy test	To confirm pregnancy
Transvaginal ultrasonography	To determine whether there is a viable intrauterine pregnancy and to evaluate for an adnexal mass or free fluid in the cul-de-sac (a molar pregnancy has a

	"snowstorm" appearance on ultrasonography)
Blood type and screen	To determine the patient's Rh status, because anti—D immune globulin should be given if the patient is Rh negative

Additional Work-Up

Quantitative β—human chorionic gonadotropin (β-hCG) measurement	Useful if an intrauterine pregnancy is not seen on ultrasound examination, in order to determine the risk of an ectopic pregnancy
	Serial β-hCG measurements are useful for determining a patient's risk of spontaneous abortion
	A gestational sac should be seen on transvaginal ultrasonogram if the β-hCG measurement is 2000 IU/L or higher; if a gestational sac is not seen, an ectopic pregnancy should be suspected
	β-hCG measurements should double over 48 hours in a viable pregnancy
Complete blood cell count	To determine whether the patient is anemic; also useful if the patient is febrile, to determine the white blood cell count
Wet-mount preparation and potassium hydroxide (KOH) microscopy of vaginal discharge	To evaluate for vaginitis
Cervical culture for *Neisseria gonorrhea* and *Chlamydia trachomatis*	If patient is at risk for a sexually transmitted disease
Pap smear	If cervical dysplasia is suspected

FURTHER READING

Beckmann CRB, Ling FW, Smith RP, et al, eds: Obstetrics and Gynecology, 5th ed. Philadelphia: Lippincott Williams & Wilkins, 2006.

Chamberlain G: Vaginal bleeding in early pregnancy—II. BMJ 1991;302:1195-1197.

Coppola PT, Coppola M: Vaginal bleeding in the first 20 weeks of pregnancy. Emerg Med Clin North Am 2003;21:667-677.

Della-Giustina D, Denny M: Ectopic pregnancy. Emerg Med Clin North Am 2003;21: 565-584.

Farquhar CM: Ectopic pregnancy. Lancet 2005;366:583-591.

Griebel CP, Halvorsen J, Golemon TB, et al: Management of spontaneous abortion. Am Fam Physician 2005;72:1243-1250.

McKennett M, Fullerton JT: Vaginal bleeding in pregnancy. Am Fam Physician 1995;51: 639-646.

Kathleen Dor

The three main causes of vaginal bleeding in the second half of
pregnancy are placenta previa, placental abruption, and preterm labor.
Placenta previa is painless, whereas placental abruption and preterm labor
are characterized by abdominal pain and uterine contractions.

Placenta previa occurs when the placenta is located close to or over
the internal cervical os. Risk factors for placenta previa include advanced
maternal age, increased parity, and prior cesarean section. The first
episode of bleeding with placenta previa usually occurs at around 30
weeks of pregnancy and is usually painless.

Placental abruption is the premature separation of the placenta. Risk
factors for placental abruption include prior abruption, abdominal trauma,
smoking, cocaine use, multiple-fetus gestation, hypertension, preeclampsia,
and thrombophilia. Placental abruption is accompanied by bleeding and
pain. It occurs in about 1% of pregnancies and is associated with significant
morbidity.

Preterm labor is defined by the onset of regular uterine contractions,
which affect cervical change and occur before the end of the 36th week
of gestation. Bloody show also is associated with labor at term.

Medications Linked to Bleeding in Middle to
Late Pregnancy

Aspirin

Clopidogrel

Heparin

Nonsteroidal anti-inflammatory drugs (NSAIDs)

Methotrexate

Misoprostol

Oxytocin

Warfarin

Causes of Vaginal Bleeding in Middle to Late Pregnancy

Cervical disease

- Cervical cancer
- Cervical erosion

- Cervical polyps
- Cervical trauma
- Cervicitis

Hematologic disorders

- Idiopathic thrombocytopenic purpura
- Leukemia
- Severe preeclampsia with thrombocytopenia
- von Willebrand disease

Labor

Medications (see previous list)

Placenta accreta

- Placenta previa
- Complete placenta previa
- Low-lying placenta previa
- Marginal placenta previa

Placental abruption

Preterm labor

Trauma

Uterine rupture

Vaginal disease

- Vaginal trauma
- Vaginitis
- Vulvar varicose veins

Vasa previa

Key Historical Features

✓ Menstrual history

✓ Estimated date of delivery

✓ Nature and amount of bleeding

✓ Presence or absence of fetal movement

✓ Loss of fluid, rupture of membranes, or both

✓ Trauma (abdominal or vaginal)

✓ Previous pregnancies and any complications, including prior placental abruptions, premature labor, or preeclampsia

✓ Previous ultrasound examinations during current pregnancy

✓ Associated pelvic, abdominal, or lower back pain, which may indicate preterm labor, labor, placental abruption, uterine rupture, pelvic inflammatory disease, or preeclampsia

✓ History of any obstetric/gynecologic surgeries or procedures, including prior cesarean sections

✓ History of any sexually transmitted diseases or pelvic inflammatory disease

✓ Medical history, especially history of bleeding disorders, thrombophilia, or hypertension

✓ Social history (smoking, alcohol use, drug use)

✓ Review of systems, especially the following:

- Fever, chills, or night sweats, which may indicate infection
- Dizziness, which may indicate a large amount of blood loss
- Headaches, which are associated with preeclampsia
- Facial or extremity swelling, which is associated with preeclampsia

Key Physical Findings

✓ Vital signs, including orthostatic assessments

✓ General evaluation of well-being

✓ If placenta previa is considered in the differential diagnosis, then ultrasonography should be performed to evaluate for placental location before a digital or speculum examination is performed, in order to prevent catastrophic bleeding

✓ If premature rupture of membranes is suspected, digital examination should be deferred until the speculum examination is performed, to evaluate for vaginal pooling

✓ If preterm labor is suspected, a test for fetal fibronectin should be performed before a digital examination

✓ Gynecologic/obstetric examination

- Perineum/vulvar examination for any lesions or trauma
- Speculum examination to evaluate for any bleeding, vaginal fluid suggestive of rupture of membranes, cervical lesions, or cervical dilatation
- Doppler ultrasonography to evaluate fetal heart rate
- Measurement of the fundal height to assess correlation with the patient's dates
- Digital examination to evaluate for cervical dilatation and effacement, as well as fetal presentation

✓ Abdominal examination for tenderness

✓ Rectal examination for hemorrhoids

✓ Skin examination for evidence of bruising, which may indicate a bleeding disorder, trauma, or abuse

Suggested Work-Up

Abdominal or transvaginal ultrasonography	To evaluate for abruption, to locate the placenta, to calculate the amniotic fluid index, to determine fetal presentation, and to determine the gestational age of the fetus
Fetal heart monitoring	To evaluate fetal well-being
External tocodynamometry	To evaluate for uterine contractions
Blood type and screen	To determine the patient's Rh status (if the patient is Rh negative, she should receive anti-D immune globulin)
Complete blood cell count (CBC)	To evaluate for anemia

Additional Work-Up

Wet-mount preparation and potassium hydroxide (KOH) microscopy of vaginal discharge	To evaluate for clue cells (bacterial vaginosis), hyphae (*Candida* infection), or *Trichomonas* infection
Group B *Streptococcus* culture	To evaluate for vaginal infection with group B streptococci so that prophylactic antibiotics can be administered if needed
Nitrazine test	If rupture of membranes is suspected (amniotic fluid is alkaline, turning nitrazine paper blue)
Fern test	If rupture of membranes is suspected (amniotic fluid, if left to dry on a slide, will have a "fern pattern")
Fetal fibronectin measurement	To evaluate the risk for preterm labor

Liver function tests, CBC, prothrombin (PT) measurement, partial thromboplastin time (PTT) measurement, assessment of fibrin split products, serum creatinine measurement, uric acid measurement, 24-hour urine measurement for creatinine clearance and protein	If preeclampsia is suspected
Betke-Kleihauer test, CBC, PT measurement, PTT measurement, assessment of fibrin split products, and fibrinogen measurement	If placental abruption is suspected
Urinalysis and urine culture	To evaluate for urinary tract infection (if preterm labor is suspected)
Cervical culture for *Neisseria gonorrhoeae* and *Chlamydia* organisms	If the patient is at risk for a sexually transmitted disease
Drug screen	If cocaine use is suspected as a cause of placental abruption
Pap smear	If cervical neoplasia is suspected or if the patient is due for cervical cancer screening

FURTHER READING

Beckmann CRB, Ling FW, Smith RP, et al, eds: Obstetrics and Gynecology, 5th ed. Philadelphia: Lippincott Williams & Wilkins, 2006.

McKennett M, Fullerton JT: Vaginal bleeding in pregnancy. Am Fam Physician 1995;51: 639-646.

Oyelese Y, Ananth CV: Placental abruption. Obstet Gynecol 2006;108:1005-1016.

Oyelese Y, Smulian J: Placenta previa, placenta accrete and vasa previa. Obstetr Gynecol 2006;107:927-941.

Toppenberg KS, Block WA: Uterine rupture: what family physicians need to know. Am Fam Physician 2002;66:823-828.

41 VAGINAL DISCHARGE

Kathleen Dor

Vaginal discharge is a common complaint of women and can either be physiologic or pathologic. Physiologic discharge is usually white or clear and thin and may have a mild odor. Accompanying symptoms such as itching, burning sensation, and redness should not be present. A woman's vaginal discharge can change with the menstrual cycle. In addition, vaginal discharge may change as a woman ages and during pregnancy.

Pathologic vaginal discharge has many different possible causes. In the United States, the two most common causes are bacterial vaginosis and candidal vaginitis. Other causes include sexually transmitted diseases, especially infections with *Chlamydia trachomatis, Neisseria gonorrhoeae*, and *Trichomonas vaginalis*.

The appropriate diagnosis of vaginal discharge is very important in order to prevent potential complications. Both bacterial vaginosis and *T. vaginalis* infection can increase the risk of preterm labor. In addition, chlamydia and gonorrhea can lead to pelvic inflammatory disease, which can result in infertility.

Medications That Can Affect Vaginal Discharge

Antibiotics (increases risk for candidiasis)

Antiseptics (may cause chemical irritation or allergic vaginitis)

Corticosteroids (increases risk for candidiasis)

Lubricants (may cause chemical irritation or allergic vaginitis)

Oral contraceptives (increase risk for candidiasis and may affect discharge as a result of estrogen effect)

Over-the-counter vaginal creams (may cause chemical irritation or allergic vaginitis)

Spermicides (may cause chemical irritation or allergic vaginitis)

Causes of Vaginal Discharge

Allergic or irritant vaginitis (deodorant, douches, spermicides, semen)

Anaerobic infections caused by foreign bodies (tampons, condoms, diaphragms)

Atrophic vaginitis

Bacterial vaginosis

Candidiasis

221

C. trachomatis

Desquamative inflammatory vaginitis

Endocervical polyp

Escherichia coli infection

Gynecologic neoplasms

Herpes simplex virus

Human immunodeficiency virus

Human papillomavirus

Intrauterine device

Medications

Mycoplasma genitalium infection

Physiologic discharge (pregnancy, menstrual cycle)

N. gonorrhoeae

Rectovaginal fistula

Staphylococcus aureus infection

Trauma

T. vaginalis

Ureaplasma urealyticum infection

Vesicovaginal fistula

Key Historical Features

✓   Duration, color, consistency, amount, and odor of discharge

✓   Associated symptoms, such as burning sensation, itching, bleeding, pelvic or abdominal pain, lesions, dysuria, or painful sexual intercourse

✓   Relation to menstrual cycle

✓   History of infertility

✓   History of gynecologic surgery

✓   History of sexually transmitted diseases or vaginitis

✓   History of abnormal Pap smear results

✓   Sexual history

✓   History of pelvic radiation therapy (which increases risk for fistula)

✓   Most recent menstrual period

✓   Use of tampons

✓   Contraceptive used (condoms, intrauterine device)

✓   Menopausal status

✓ Medical history

- History of diabetes or symptoms of diabetes (which increases risk of candidal infections)
- History of human immunodeficiency virus (HIV) infection
- History of inflammatory bowel disease (IBD) or symptoms of IBD (which increases risk for fistula)

✓ Obstetric history, including history of obstetric trauma (increases risk for fistula)

✓ Surgical history

✓ Medications, including over-the-counter medications

Key Physical Findings

✓ Vital signs, especially assessment for the presence of fever

✓ External genital examination

- Examination of the vulva, which may appear erythematous with candidal or *T. vaginalis* infection
- Examination for satellite lesions, which may be seen with candidal infection
- Examination for ulcerative lesions, which may be seen with herpes simplex

✓ Speculum examination

- Examination of the vagina, which may appear erythematous with candidal or *T. vaginalis* infection
- Inspection for foreign bodies or neoplastic lesions
- Examination for "strawberry" cervix (punctate hemorrhages), which may be seen with *T. vaginalis* infection

✓ Appearance of discharge

- Frothy, thin, yellow/green discharge, which is consistent with *T. vaginalis* infection
- Thick white discharge, which is consistent with candidal infection
- Thin, grayish-white discharge, which is consistent with bacterial vaginosis
- Mucopurulent or purulent cervical discharge, which is suggestive of chlamydia, gonorrhea, or herpes simplex
- Mucopurulent or purulent urethral discharge, which is suggestive of chlamydia or gonorrhea
- Thin, clear, or bloody discharge, which is suggestive of atrophic vaginitis

✓ Odor of discharge
  - Fishy odor, which is suggestive of bacterial vaginosis
  - Foul odor, which may be caused by *T. vaginalis* or by anaerobic infections as a result of forgotten foreign bodies
✓ Bimanual examination to evaluate for cervical motion or uterine or adnexal tenderness, which is suggestive of pelvic inflammatory disease

Suggested Work-Up

Microscopy includes the following tests:

Wet-mount preparation of cervical discharge	To detect trichomonads (trichomonas) or clue cells (bacterial vaginosis), polymorphonuclear leukocytes (a ratio of polymorphonuclear leukocytes to epithelial cells greater than 1:1 is seen with *T. vaginalis* infection, gonorrhea, chlamydia, and herpes simplex), or round parabasal cells (which are seen with atrophic vaginitis)
Potassium hydroxide (KOH) preparation	To detect candidal infections (pseudohyphae or budding yeast)
Whiff test	To detect bacterial vaginosis (fishy odor with KOH)
Measurement of pH	A pH greater than 4 could indicate bacterial vaginosis or *T. vaginalis* infection (normal vaginal pH is 3.8 to 4.2)
Pap smear	To evaluate for cervical dysplasia
Endocervical swab or urine nucleic acid amplification test for *Chlamydia* organisms and *N. gonorrhoeae* (endocervical swab or urine)	To detect infections by these organisms

Additional Work-Up

Urine pregnancy test	If pregnancy is suspected
Sabouraud medium or Nickerson agar culture	To evaluate for candidal infections if the diagnosis is unclear

Diamond medium culture or polymerase chain reaction (PCR) testing	To evaluate for *T. vaginalis* infection if the diagnosis is suspected and wet-mount test is negative
Gram stain of cervical discharge	For the presence of intracellular gram-negative diplococci, which indicates gonorrhea, if an immediate diagnosis is needed
Viral culture of herpetic lesions	If herpes simplex infection is suspected
Biopsy	To evaluate lesions that appear to be neoplastic
Colposcopy	To evaluate suspicious lesions on the cervix
Thayer-Martin agar culture of cervical discharge	To evaluate for gonorrhea
HIV test	If the patient is at risk for HIV infection
Chlamydia culture of cervical discharge	If chlamydial infection is suspected

FURTHER READING

Egan ME, Lipsky MS: Diagnosis of vaginitis. Am Fam Physician 2000;62:1095-1104.

Fox KK, Behets F: Vaginal discharge: how to pinpoint the cause. Postgrad Med 1995;989: 87-104.

Henn EW, Kruger TF, Siebert TI: Vaginal discharge reviewed: the adult pre-menopausal female. S Afr Fam Pract 2005;47(2):30-31, 34-38.

Mitchell H: Vaginal discharge—causes, diagnosis, and treatment. BMJ 2004;328:1306-1308.

Owen MK, Clenney TL: Management of vaginitis. Am Fam Physician 2004;70:2125-2132.

Kathleen Dor

Vulvar pruritus can be caused by a number of different conditions ranging from localized diseases to systemic diseases. The age of the woman is very important in the differential diagnosis. In premenopausal women, contact dermatitis, lichen simplex, and candidal vaginitis are common causes of vulvar pruritus. In postmenopausal women, common causes include atrophic vaginitis, lichen sclerosis, vulvar intraepithelial neoplasia, and vulvar cancer. In patients with diabetes, candidal infections are prevalent.

It is often very difficult to diagnose the cause of vulvar lesions. If the diagnosis is unclear, a biopsy should be performed in order to evaluate for malignancy. Most vulvar cancers occur in postmenopausal women; about 10% of these malignancies occur in younger women.

Medications Linked to Vulvar Pruritus

Amoxicillin–clavulanic acid (can cause cholestasis)

Anabolic steroids (can cause cholestasis)

Erythromycin (can cause cholestasis)

Oral contraceptives (can cause cholestasis)

Penicillin (can cause allergic reaction)

Phenothiazines (can cause cholestasis)

Sulfa medications (can cause allergic reaction)

Tamoxifen

Topical medications/over-the-counter products:

- Anesthetics
- Antibiotics
- Antifungal creams
- Antihistamines
- Disinfectants
- Estrogen creams
- Lubricants
- Spermicides

Causes of Vulvar Pruritus

Adenomatous polyps

Allergic contact dermatitis

Anal fissure

Atopic dermatitis

Atrophic vaginitis

Bacterial vaginosis

Breast cancer

Carcinoid syndrome

Cloacogenic carcinoma

Diabetes

Fistulas

Fox-Fordyce disease

Gastric cancer

Genital warts

Hemorrhoids

Herpes

Histiocytosis X

Human immunodeficiency virus (HIV) infection

Hodgkin disease

Hyperthyroidism

Hypothyroidism

Inflammatory bowel disease

Intertrigo

Iron deficiency anemia

Irritant contact dermatitis

Leukemia

Lichen planus

Lichen sclerosis

Lichen simplex chronicus

Liver disease or biliary disease

Lung cancer

Lymphoma

Molluscum contagiosum

Multiple myeloma

Mycosis fungoides

Pediculosis pubis

Polycythemia vera

Proctitis

Psoriasis

Rectal, anal, or colon cancer

Renal failure or uremia

Scabies

Seborrheic dermatitis

Squamous cell hyperplasia

Tinea cruris

Trichomonas

Vulvovaginal candidiasis

Vulvar intraepithelial neoplasia

Vulvar carcinoma

Key Historical Features

✓ Constitutional symptoms

- Associated symptoms that may suggest a systemic disease, such as fatigue (caused by malignancy, renal failure, thyroid disease, iron deficiency anemia), unintentional weight loss (caused by diabetes, malignancy), or jaundice (caused by biliary or liver disease)

✓ Gynecologic symptoms and history

- Menopausal status
- Location, duration, and severity of pruritus
- Association of pruritus with menses
- Associated symptoms such as pain, lesions, or vaginal discharge
- Sexual history
- History of sexually transmitted diseases
- History of prior vulvar or gynecologic diseases
- Association with common irritants: medications (see previous list), body fluids, tampons, sanitary napkins, condoms, shaving, waxing, douching, soaps, detergents, clothing dyes, bubble bath, or overzealous cleansing

✓ Gastrointestinal symptoms

- Diarrhea, which may indicate inflammatory bowel disease
- Rectal bleeding, which may indicate colon cancer

✓ Medical history, especially history of diabetes, thyroid disease, renal disease, liver disease, or malignancy

Key Physical Findings

✓ Examination of the vulva for lesions (note color, texture, location)

- Lichen simplex chronicus, which manifests with diffusely erythematous areas

- Lichen planus, which manifests with red ulcerated lesions with white lacy bands
- Psoriasis, which manifests with raised lesions with a silver scale and an erythematous base
- Seborrheic dermatitis, which manifests with symmetric reddish-yellowish lesions with an oily crust, sparing the labia minora
- Lichen sclerosis, which manifests with thin whitish areas of epithelium
- Vulvar intraepithelial neoplasia, which has a variable presentation: white, red, or pigmented lesions that may be an isolated patch or extensive
- Vulvar carcinoma, which has a variable presentation: red or white ulcer or exophytic lesion, usually on the labia majora
- *Candida* infection, which manifests with red lesions with satellite lesions
- Tinea cruris, which manifests with raised edges and well-demarcated lesions
- Squamous cell hyperplasia, which manifests with areas of thickened epithelium (usually of the clitoris and labia majora)

✓ Speculum examination to evaluate the vagina and cervix for discharge, lesions, or erythema

✓ Examination of the perianal area for any lesions

Suggested Work-Up

Scrapings for fungal culture and microscopy	To evaluate for tinea cruris
Wet-mount preparation of vaginal secretions	To evaluate for bacterial vaginosis or *Trichomonas vaginalis* infection
Potassium hydroxide (KOH) preparation of vaginal secretions	To evaluate for *Candida* infection
Colposcopy	To evaluate for vulvar atypia
Biopsy	If the diagnosis is unclear or if neoplasia is suspected

Additional Work-Up

Patch testing	If contact dermatitis is suspected
Serum bilirubin measurement	If biliary disease is suspected

Liver function tests	If liver disease is suspected
Complete blood cell count	If a hematologic disorder is suspected
Serum creatinine measurement	If kidney disease is suspected
HIV test	If HIV infection is suspected or the patient is at risk
Thyroid-stimulating hormone (TSH) measurement	If thyroid disease is suspected
Fasting blood glucose measurement	If diabetes is suspected
Viral culture	To evaluate for herpes if ulcerative lesions are present
Colonoscopy or sigmoidoscopy	If a colonic cause is suspected

FURTHER READING

Bohl TG: Overview of vulvar pruritis through the life cycle. Clin Obstet Gynecol 2005;48:786-807.

Bornstein J, Pascal B, Abramovich H: The common problem of vulvar pruritus. Obstet Gynecol Surv 1993;48(2):111-118.

Moses S: Pruritus. Am Fam Physician 2003;68:1135-1142.

Welsh B, Howard A, Cook K: Vulval itch. Austral Fam Physician 2004;33:505-510.

Theodore O'Connell

Clinically significant weight loss can be defined as the loss of 10 pounds (4.5 kg) or more than 5% of the usual body weight over 6 to 12 months, especially when the weight loss is progressive. Weight loss greater than 10% in that amount of time represents protein-energy malnutrition, which is associated with impaired physiologic function, such as impaired cell-mediated and humoral immunity. Weight loss greater than 20% in the same time represents severe protein-energy malnutrition and is associated with organ dysfunction.

Dieting and eating disorders, such as anorexia nervosa and bulimia nervosa, account for most cases of intentional weight loss. Unintentional weight loss can be divided into four problems: anorexia, dysphagia, weight loss despite normal intake, or socioeconomic problems.

Malignancies account for approximately one third of all patients with unintentional weight loss. Gastrointestinal disorders are the most common nonmalignant organic causes in patients with unintentional weight loss, accounting for about 15% of cases. Medications are a frequently overlooked potential cause of unintentional weight loss, particularly in elderly patients. Adverse effects of medications, such as anorexia, nausea, diarrhea, dysphagia, and dysgeusia, may alter the intake, absorption, and use of nutrients.

Weight loss occurs commonly in elderly individuals. Among noninstitutionalized elderly persons, depression, cancer, and benign gastrointestinal tract diseases are the most common causes of weight loss. Among nursing home residents, psychiatric and neurologic illnesses account for the greatest proportion of weight loss.

In most patients, the cause of unintentional weight loss may be identified through a detailed history and physical examination. The first step in evaluating a complaint of weight loss is quantifying the weight loss. The symptoms documented from the history can guide the clinician to one of the four causal categories: anorexia, dysphagia, weight loss despite normal intake, and social factors. The suggested laboratory evaluation is outlined later in this chapter. Additional testing should be directed by findings from the history, physical examination, or initial laboratory evaluation. Patients with normal physical examination and laboratory findings are unlikely to have a serious physical illness.

Medications Associated with Weight Loss

Angiotensin-converting enzyme (ACE) inhibitors

Alendronate

Allopurinol

Amantadine

Amphetamines

Antibiotics

- Atovaquone
- Ciprofloxacin
- Clarithromycin
- Doxycycline
- Ethambutol
- Griseofulvin
- Metronidazole
- Ofloxacin
- Pentamidine
- Rifabutin
- Tetracycline

Anticholinergics

Anticonvulsants

Antihistamines

Benzodiazepines

Bisphosphonates

Calcium channel blockers

Carbamazepine

Chemotherapeutic agents

Clonidine

Corticosteroids

Decongestants

Digoxin

Dopamine agonists

Gold

Hormone replacement therapy

Hydralazine

Hydrochlorothiazide

Iron

Levodopa

Lithium

Metformin

Methimazole

Neuroleptics

Nicotine

Nitroglycerin

Nonsteroidal anti-inflammatory drugs (NSAIDs)

Opiates

Penicillamine

Pergolide

Phenytoin

Potassium

Propranolol

Quinidine

Selective serotonin reuptake inhibitors

Selegiline

Spironolactone

Statins

Theophylline

Tricyclic antidepressants

Causes of Weight Loss

Alcoholism

Cardiovascular disease

- Congestive heart failure
- Mesenteric ischemia

Cocaine use

Dietary factors (low-salt, low-cholesterol diets)

Endocrine disorders

- Adrenal insufficiency
- Diabetes mellitus
- Hyperparathyroidism
- Hyperthyroidism
- Hypothyroidism
- Panhypopituitarism
- Pheochromocytoma

Gastrointestinal disease

- Atrophic gastritis
- Celiac disease
- Cholelithiasis

- Chronic pancreatitis
- Constipation
- Diarrhea
- Dysphagia (oropharyngeal or esophageal)
- Gastroparesis
- Inflammatory bowel disease
- Malabsorption resulting from bacterial overgrowth, pancreatic exocrine deficiency, or celiac disease
- Peptic ulcer disease
- Pseudo-obstruction
- Reflux esophagitis

Inability to feed self

Infections

- Fungal disease
- Human immunodeficiency virus (HIV) infection
- Parasites
- Subacute bacterial endocarditis
- Tuberculosis

Malignancies

- Breast
- Gastrointestinal
- Genitourinary
- Hepatobiliary
- Hematologic
- Lung
- Ovarian

Medications

Neurologic disease

- Cerebrovascular accident
- Delirium
- Dementia
- Multiple sclerosis
- Parkinson disease
- Quadriplegia
- Tardive dyskinesia

Nutritional disorders

Oral factors

- Periodontal disease

- Poor dentition
- Xerostomia

Pulmonary disease

- Chronic obstructive pulmonary disease

Psychiatric disorders

- Anorexia nervosa
- Anxiety disorders
- Bulimia nervosa
- Depression
- Paranoia

Renal disease

- Hemodialysis
- Nephrotic syndrome
- Uremia

Rheumatologic disease

- Giant cell arteritis
- Scleroderma

Socioeconomic conditions

Swallowing disorders

Visual impairments

Key Historical Features

✓ Amount of weight loss

✓ Determination of whether the patient predominantly is not hungry, is nauseated after meals, has difficulty eating or swallowing, or has functional or social problems that may be interfering with the ability to obtain or enjoy food

✓ Presence of indigestion or reflux symptoms

✓ Abdominal pain

✓ Changes in bowel habits

✓ For geriatric patients, interviewing a knowledgeable caretaker

✓ Dietary history

- Availability of food
- Use of nutritional or herbal supplements
- Amount of food consumed
- Adequacy of the patient's diet
- Daily caloric intake

✓ Discussion of functional and mental status

✓ Medical history, especially history of previous gastrointestinal conditions

✓ Surgical history, especially history of previous gastrointestinal surgery

✓ Medications

✓ Social history

- Financial situation
- Lifestyle
- Living arrangements and home environment
- Occupation
- Support network
- Travel
- Use of transportation

✓ Thorough review of systems

Key Physical Findings

✓ Vital signs

✓ Height, weight, and body mass index

✓ Examination of the oral cavity

✓ Cardiopulmonary examination

✓ Abdominal examination

✓ Rectal examination

✓ Mental status examination and formal cognitive testing with an instrument such as the Folstein Mini-Mental State Examination

✓ Evaluation for depression with an instrument such as the PHQ-9 (nine-item depression scale of the Patient Health Questionnaire) or the Geriatric Depression Scale

✓ Examination of the nervous system

✓ Functional assessment, including evaluations of sight, hearing, gait, and self-care ability (tools include the Katz scale of activities of daily living and the Lawton scale of instrumental activities of daily living)

Suggested Work-Up

Complete blood cell count (CBC)	To evaluate for infection, anemia, or lymphoproliferative disorder

Chemistry panel	To evaluate for diabetes mellitus, dehydration, or renal dysfunction
Thyroid-stimulating hormone measurement	To evaluate for hypothyroidism or hyperthyroidism
Urinalysis	To evaluate for infection, renal dysfunction, or dehydration
Fecal occult blood test	To screen for gastrointestinal malignancy
Chest radiography	To evaluate for infection, malignancy, or cardiopulmonary disease
Upper endoscopy or upper gastrointestinal series	Should be considered in patients with anorexia, absence of other symptoms, and persistent weight loss, because peptic ulcer disease and gastroesophageal reflux may be clinically silent

Additional Work-Up

Measurement of erythrocyte sedimentation rate	To evaluate for inflammatory processes
Blood culture	If infection is suspected
Purified protein derivative (PPD) test	If tuberculosis is suspected
HIV test	If risk factors are present or if HIV infection is suspected
Rapid plasma reagin (RPR)	If risk factors for syphilis are present or if physical findings suggest the presence of syphilis infection
Growth hormone measurement	To evaluate for endocrine deficiency
Sigmoidoscopy or colonoscopy	If a colonic lesion is suspected
Computed tomographic (CT) scanning	Low yield but possibly helpful in diagnosing malignancy, abscess, chronic pancreatitis, intestinal complications, and so forth

| Measurement of serum prealbumin, transferrin, and albumin | Not useful in determining the cause of weight loss, but possibly useful in guiding supplement selection |

FURTHER READING

Alibhai SM, Greenwood C, Payette H: An approach to the management of unintentional weight loss in elderly people. CMAJ 2005;172:773-780.

Bouras EP, Lange SM, Scolapio JS: Rational approach to patients with unintentional weight loss. Mayo Clin Proc 2001;76:923-929.

Gazewood JD, Mehr DR: Diagnosis and management of weight loss in the elderly. J Fam Pract 1998;47:19-25.

Huffman GB: Evaluating and treating unintentional weight loss in the elderly. Am Fam Physician 2002;65:640-650.

Robertson RG, Montagnini M: Geriatric failure to thrive. Am Fam Physician 2004;70: 343-350.

Index

Note: Page numbers followed by b indicate boxed material; f, figures, t, tables.